Blood Type O- Negative Cook Book For Beginners

A Guide to Nourishing Your Health And Living Your Best Life As A Universal Donor With Over 100 Delicious Expert Recipes.

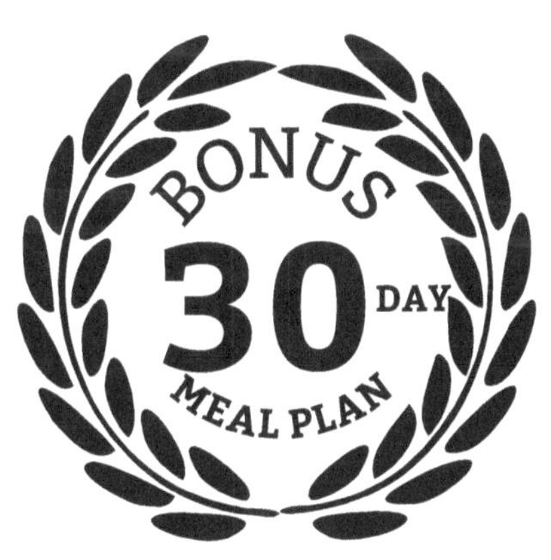

By MARY MAAG

I

II

DISCLAIMER❗

This is a work of nonfiction. The recipes, advice, and details are derived from the author's personal experiences and research. Although every effort has been taken to ensure the accuracy of the content, the publisher and author expressly disclaim all warranties, including implied warranties of fitness for a particular purpose, and make no representations or warranties concerning the correctness or completeness of the contents of this work.

The author does not advocate or recommend any particular brands, goods, or services mentioned in this book.

Before adopting any major dietary or lifestyle changes based on the advice in this book, the reader should speak with a healthcare provider before implementing any major dietary or lifestyle modifications based on the advice in this book.

Regarding any harm or loss caused or alleged to be caused either directly or indirectly by the material in this book, the publisher and author shall have no obligation or duty to any person or entity.

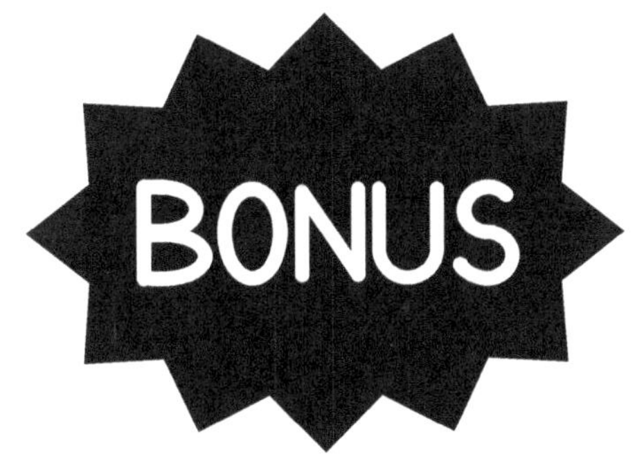

Here is Your 30-Day Meal Plan

All Recipes Are in This Book

Use The Tick Box To Keep Track

DAY 1

☐ **Breakfast**
Scrambled Eggs with Zucchini

☐ **Lunch**
Baked Falafel

☐ **Dinner**
Fish Tacos

DAY 2

☐ **Breakfast**
Omelette with Vegetables

☐ **Lunch**
Lamb meatball

☐ **Dinner**
Lemon Ginger Salmon

DAY 3

☐ **Breakfast**
Smoked Salmon and Avocado Toast

☐ **Lunch**
Asian Beef and Broccoli Stir-Fry

☐ **Dinner**
Spring pesto pasta

DAY 4

☐ **Breakfast**
Quinoa Breakfast Bowl

☐ **Lunch**
Tomato Greek salad

☐ **Dinner**
Shrimp and Veggie Skewers with Quinoa Tabbouleh

DAY 5

☐ **Breakfast**
Spinach and Mushroom Frittata

☐ **Lunch**
Pizza Salad

☐ **Dinner**
Lasagna

DAY 6

☐ **Breakfast**
Brown Rice Pancake

☐ **Lunch**
Salmon Quinoa Bowl

☐ **Dinner**
Moroccan Lamb Tagine

DAY 7

☐ **Breakfast**
Cherry Scones

☐ **Lunch**
Adzuki Sandwich

☐ **Dinner**
Turkey and Vegetable Stir-Fry with Brown Rice

DAY 8

☐ **Breakfast**
Broccoli Feta Frittata

☐ **Lunch**
Grilled Chicken Salad

☐ **Dinner**
Pasta Carbonara with Crispy Kale

DAY 9

☐ **Breakfast**
Pear Rosemary Bread

☐ **Lunch**
Shrimp and Avocado Sushi Bowls

☐ **Dinner**
Spicy seafood

DAY 10

☐ **Breakfast**
Maple Sausage Scramble

☐ **Lunch**
Grilled Veggie and Hummus Wrap

☐ **Dinner**
Baked Salmon with Quinoa and Steamed Asparagus

CONTINUE

PAGE 263

ABOUT MARY MAAG

Mary Maag is an utterly devoted and caring dietitian who's determined to motivate and direct people toward living a balanced and wholesome life. With an intense enthusiasm for nutrition and a pledge to promote healthy habits. Mary contributes abundant skill to her position as a dependable well-being supporter. She has invested years refining her abilities and understanding in the nutrition field. Her professional path is characterized by a tireless quest for fact-based practices and an authentic wish to enable people to make knowledgeable decisions regarding their health.

In addition to her professional endeavours, Mary embraces a family-focused way of life. As a caring wife and mother, she comprehends the intricacies of managing a hectic household while emphasising health. Her personal experiences as a parent highlight the practicality of her counsel and make her an approachable guide for families striving for a more healthful way of life.

Mary's advocacy extends further than standard dietary recommendations. She values thinking about people's whole wellness and their families' well-being. Her method combines nutrition, awareness, and practical advice for fostering a balanced and maintainable way of life. "Blood Type O- Negative Cook-Book for Beginners" shows Mary's dedication to imparting her know-how to a wider audience. In this book, she adeptly integrates her professional understanding with a true wish to positively impact her readers' lives.

CONTENTS TABLE

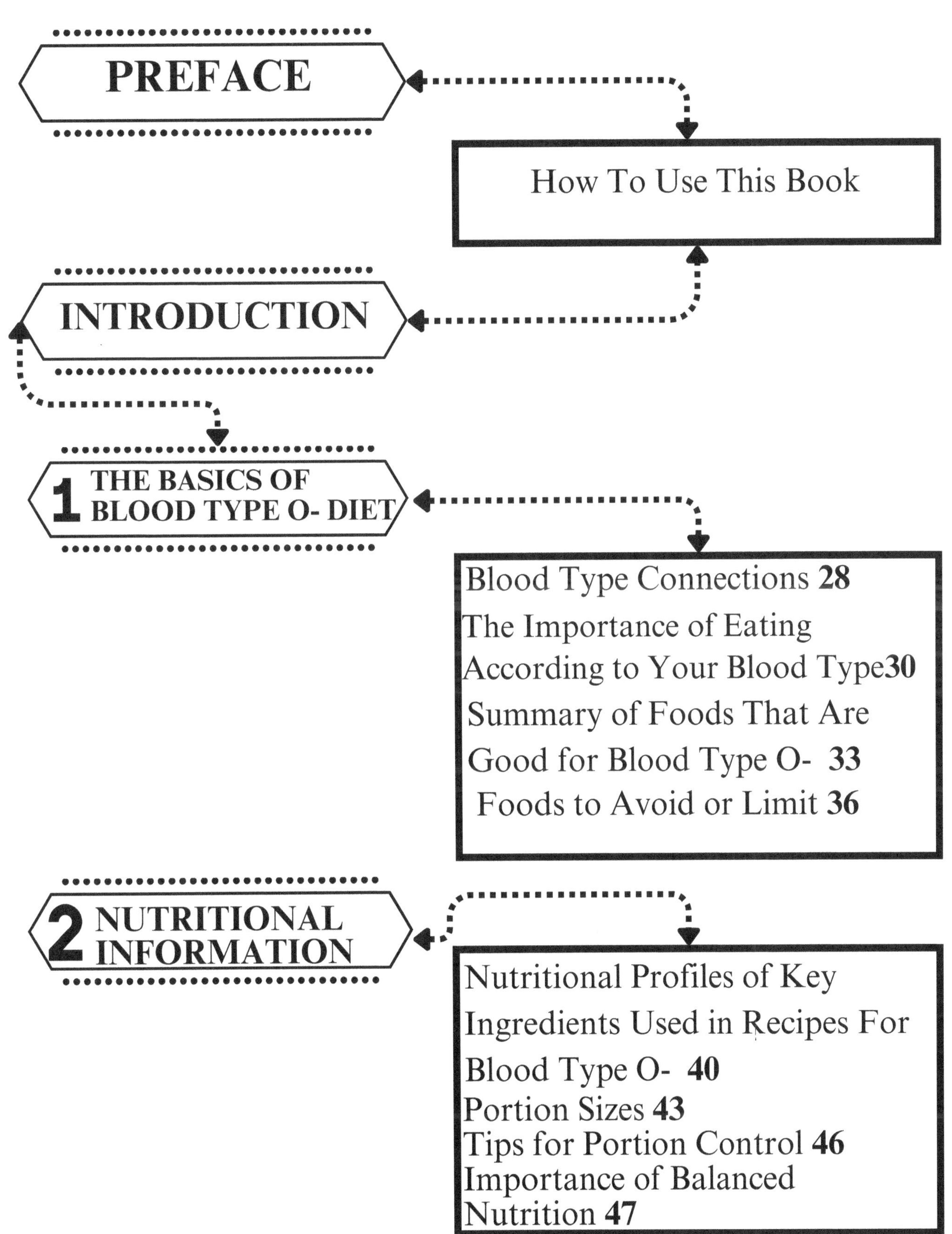

PREFACE

How To Use This Book

INTRODUCTION

1 THE BASICS OF BLOOD TYPE O- DIET

Blood Type Connections **28**

The Importance of Eating According to Your Blood Type **30**

Summary of Foods That Are Good for Blood Type O- **33**

Foods to Avoid or Limit **36**

2 NUTRITIONAL INFORMATION

Nutritional Profiles of Key Ingredients Used in Recipes For Blood Type O- **40**

Portion Sizes **43**

Tips for Portion Control **46**

Importance of Balanced Nutrition **47**

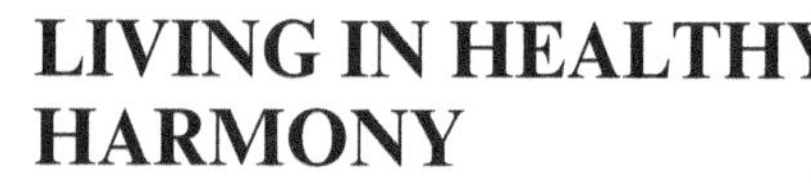

LIVING IN HEALTHY HARMONY

Exercise Choices for Blood Type O- Individuals **55**

The Role of Good Rest In Ultimate Health **60**

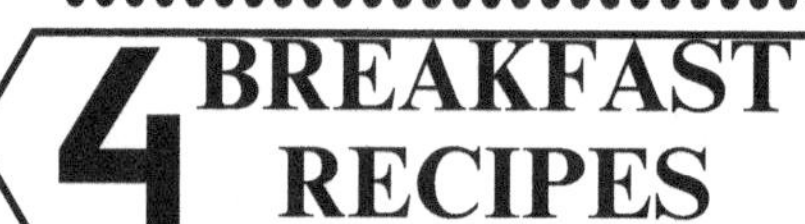

4 BREAKFAST RECIPES

Scrambled eggs with spinach and turkey bacon **66**

Omelette with Vegetables **68**

Smoked Salmon and Avocado Toast **70**

Quinoa Breakfast Bowl **72**

Spinach and Mushroom Frittata **74**

Brown Rice Pancake **76**

Cherry Scones **78**

Broccoli Feta Frittata **80**

Pear Rosemary Bread **82**

Maple Sausage Scramble **84**

5 LUNCH RECIPES

Baked Falafel **88**

Lamb Meatball **90**

Asian Beef &Broccoli Stir-Fry **92**

Tomato Greek Salad **94**

Pizza Salad **96**

Salmon Quinoa Bowl **98**

Adzuki Bean Meatballs **100**

Grilled Chicken Salad **102**

Shrimp and Avocado Sushi Bowls **104**

Grilled Veggie and Hummus Wrap **106**

6 DINNER RECIPES

Fish Tacos **110**

Lemon ginger Salmon **112**

Spring pesto pasta **114**

Shrimp and Veggie Skewers with Quinoa Tabbouleh **116**

Lasagna **118**

Moroccan Lamb Tagine **120**

Turkey and Vegetable Stir-Fry with Brown Rice **122**

Pasta Carbonara with Crispy Kale **124**

Spicy Seafood **126**

Baked Salmon with Quinoa and Steamed Asparagus **128**

7 VEGAN RECIPES

Vegan Lentil Shepherd's Pie **132**

Vegan Lentil Sloppy Joes **136**

Vegan Chickpea Curry **140**

Quinoa & Black Bean Chili **142**

Healthy Lentil Tacos **144**

Buddha Bowl with Shredded sprouts **146**

Miso Soup with Crispy Smoked Tofu **148**

8 VEGETARIAN RECIPES

Vegetarian Butternut Squash **152**

French Onion Soup **154**

Roasted Root Vegetables **156**

Slow Cooker Dahl **158**

Slow Cooker Oat **160**

Leek Fritter **162**

Mozzarella Sticks with Spicy Dipping **164**

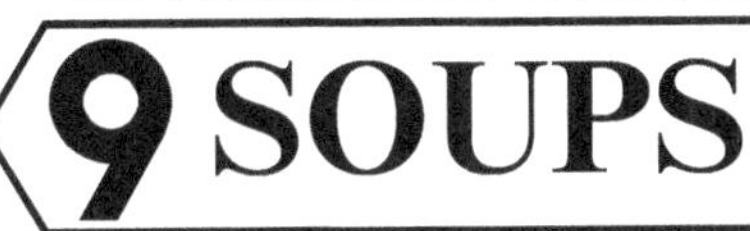

9 SOUPS

Tomato Basil Soup **168**
Parsnip Soup **170**
Turkey Chili **172**
Quinoa Herbed Soup **174**
Spicy Collards **176**
Brussels Soup **178**
Turkey and Kale Soup **180**
Pumpkin Soup **182**
Curried Okra soup **184**
Butternut Soup **186**

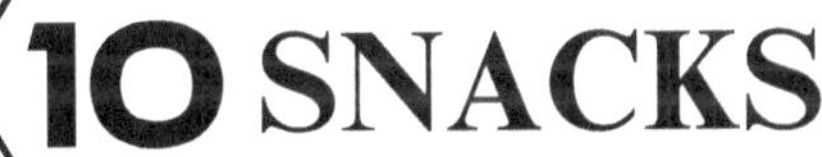

10 SNACKS

Baked Grapefruits **190**
Cucumber Slices with Tzatziki **192**
Mozzarella marinade **194**
Healthy pizza **196**
Rice cake **198**
Carrot Sticks with Hummus **200**
Apple chips **202**
Apple pie **204**
Almond Butter and Apple Slices **208**
Seaweed Snacks **209**

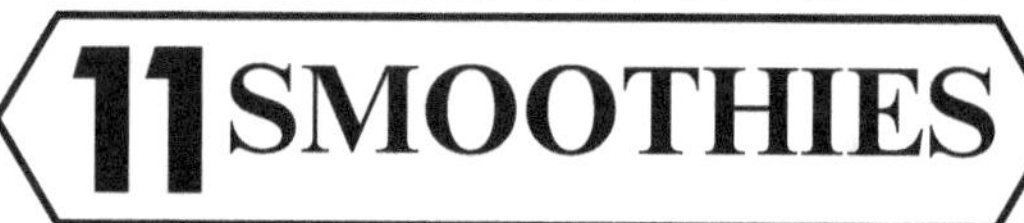

11 SMOOTHIES

Cherry Almond Smoothie **212**

Banana Almond Smoothie **213**

Tropical Paradise Smoothie **214**

Green Goddess Smoothie **215**

Pineapple Coconut Smoothie **216**

Minty Matcha Smoothie **217**

Cherry Almond Smoothie **218**

12 BEVERAGES

Green Juice **220**
Kale Juice **221**
Turmeric Latte **222**
Matcha Tea **223**
Cucumber Mint Cooler **224**
Berry Juice **225**
Watermelon Mint Refresher **226**

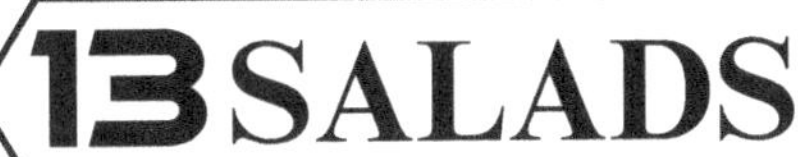 13 SALADS

Caprese Salad **228**

Tuna Nicoise Salad **229**

Greek Salad **230**

Asian Sesame Chicken Salad **231**

Mediterranean Quinoa Salad **232**

Avocado Shrimp Salad **233**

Grilled Chicken Caesar Salad **234**

14 SAUCES AND CONDIMENTS

Chimichurri Sauce **236**
Sesame Ginger Sauce **237**
Coconut Curry Sauce **238**
Avocado Cream Sauce **239**
Roasted Red Pepper Sauce **240**
Basil Pesto **241**
Balsamic Glaze **242**
Tzatziki Sauce **243**
Sriracha Mayo **244**
Guacamole **245**

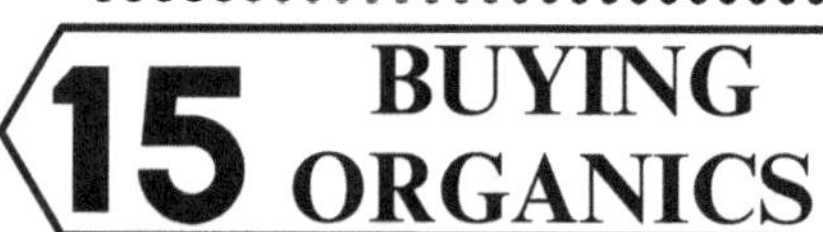

15 BUYING ORGANICS

How to Identify Organic Produce

Types of organic labels 249

Guide for Shopping Organic Produce 251

Benefits of Choosing Organic Foods for Blood Type O-

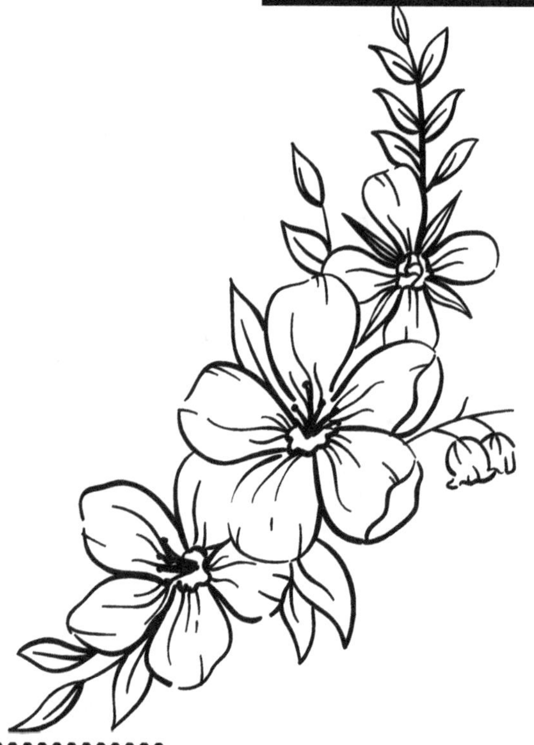

16 STORING FOOD SAFELY 000

Advice for Food Preservation **256**

Reducing Food Wastage **259**

17 CONCLUSION

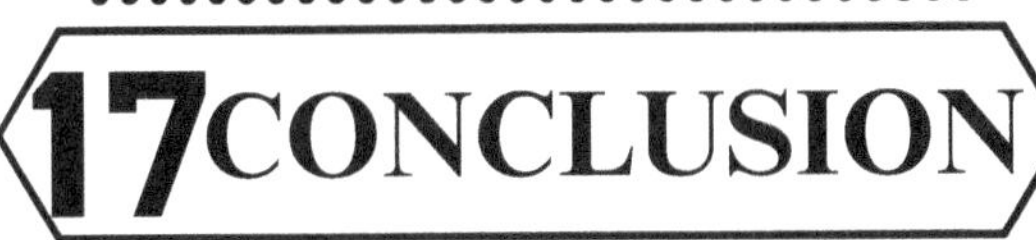

CONCLUSION

266

Act Now and Document Your Culinary Journey

This page was intentionally left blank.

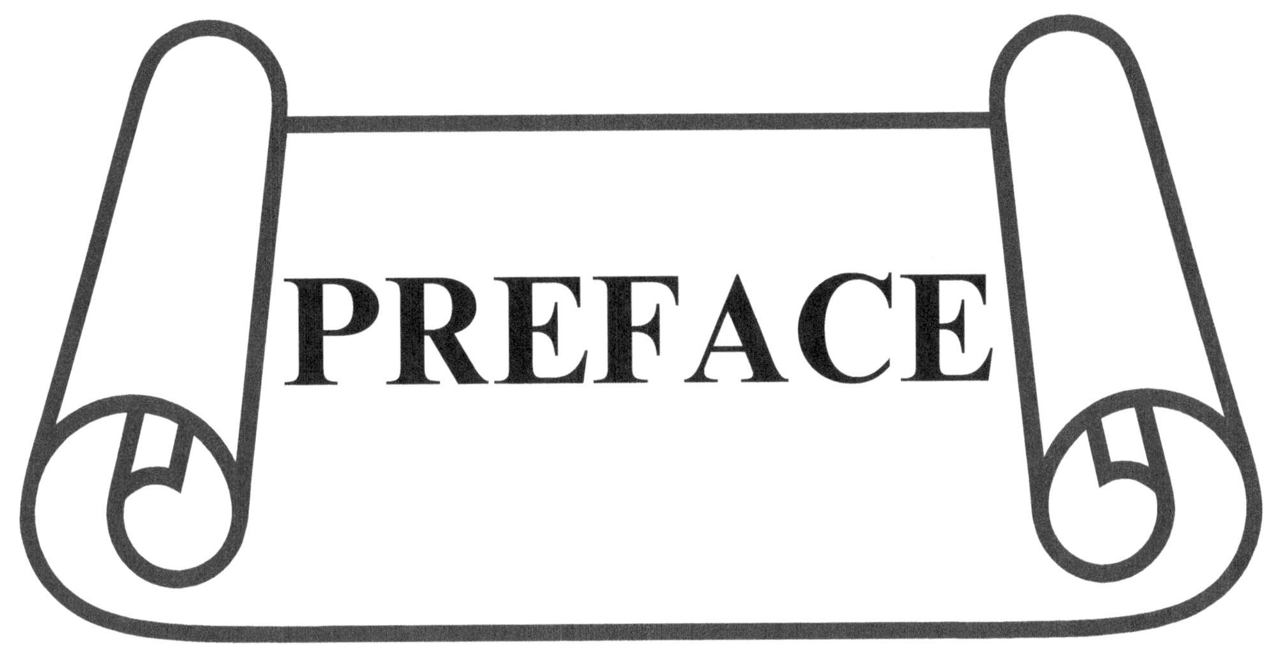

As the saying goes, "Your food could be your medicine or it could be your poison". Countless research and discoveries throughout history concerning the connections between the type of food you eat and your health have been made. The fascinating thing is that only a few seem to pay attention to the overall body's internal environment and how the type of food we ingest inside affects our health either positively or negatively. Consider it this way, it is not all crops that can grow in some specific soils. No matter the kind of fertilizers you apply to it, it struggles since it is not the ideal environment to express itself well as a crop. The idea of blood type diets has become more popular recently, providing a customary meal plan based on the blood type of a person and their internal body environment. As an O- (negative) individual, you are a universal donor because you have a unique genetic composition that affects how your body reacts to certain nutritional food.

The purpose of this cookbook is to give people with blood type O- (negative) the ability to make enlightened food decisions that will help them maintain vibrant health and energy. With the help of deep research through historical nutritional patterns, professional advice, advanced cooking techniques, and the blood type O- (negative) diet's principles, I've put together a selection of more than 100 flavorful meals that will fuel your distinctive body.

This book provides an easy-to-use guide to sticking with the blood type O- (negative) diet's principles and also leading you towards your best life possible. This isn't just a list of recipes, it is so much more. The following pages contain the following information:

- A comprehensive introduction to the fundamentals of the blood type O-negative diet, covering the background of blood type evolution and the ideas behind Mendelian genetics.

- Professionally crafted recipes for breakfast, lunch, dinner, snacks, desserts, and more, all well planned to comply with blood type O- negative specific dietary guidelines.

- Nutritional data are made available for every recipe, offering insightful information on macronutrient contents, calorie counts, and important vitamins and minerals. Prep time, cook time and servings are also included because I believe you value and work with your time very well.

- From ingredient replacements to storage suggestions, useful hints and techniques are all included to improve your culinary experience.

This cookbook is your reliable guide to the best possible health and well-being, regardless of your experience level with blood type diets.

How to use this book as a Beginner

To ensure you get the most out of this cookbook, here's a quick guide:

- **Introduction:** The introduction provides an overview of Mendel's rules and a synopsis of the evolution of blood types. You can better appreciate the recipes and dietary suggestions that follow if you grasp these fundamental ideas.

- **Knowing Your Blood Type**: Spend some time learning about the fundamentals of the blood type O- diet if you're not familiar with the idea of blood type diets. Learn how your blood type affects the foods you eat and why some foods are better avoided while others are advised.

- **Getting Around the Recipes:** The cookbook is broken up into chapters that concentrate on various food groups and meal categories. There's a wide range of recipes to try, so you can find inspiration for breakfasts, lunches, or delectable desserts.

- **Recipe Selection:** Look through the recipes and select the ones that fit your dietary requirements and taste preferences. Each recipe is created with skill to provide mouthwatering flavors and filling meals that are in line with the guidelines of the blood type O– diet.

- **Ingredients and Instructions:** Before you start cooking, carefully go over the ingredients and directions for each recipe. To ensure good results, pay attention to any unique cooking methods or techniques.

- **Customization:** You are welcome to alter the recipes to fit your specific dietary requirements and personal preferences. To customize meals that are most effective for you, you can change the ingredients, adjust the seasonings, or alter the portion sizes.

- **Nutritional Information:** Take advantage of the nutritional information provided for each recipe, including calorie counts, macronutrient breakdowns, and key vitamins and minerals. This information can help you make informed choices about your diet and ensure that you're meeting your nutritional needs.

- **Cooking Tips and Tricks:** Throughout the cookbook, you'll find helpful tips and tricks to enhance your cooking experience. From storage suggestions to ingredient substitutions, these insights will empower you to become a more confident and skilled home cook.

- **Share Your Experience:** If you try a recipe from the cookbook, I'd love to hear about your experience! Share your feedback or Review with me on Amazon to enable me to serve you better.

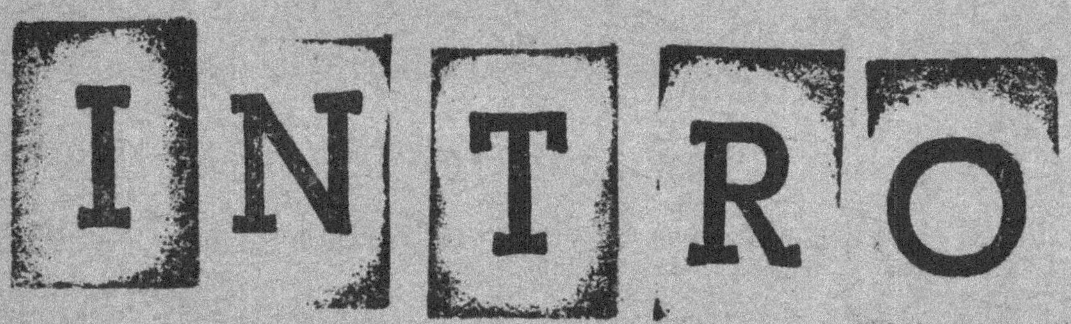

INTRODUCTION

It was Thanksgiving day, my husband, the children and I decided we would share it with those at the hospital for one reason or another, especially the ones whose family members are not around or those who do not have anyone at all. We were able to put smiles on the faces of some of those patients.

While at the hospital we experienced an emergency situation of a patient who was involved in a fatal auto crash and had lost a huge amount of blood and needed an immediate blood transfusion. She was blood type AB- (negative). All efforts to get the required amount of pint needed proved abortive, it was a matter of life and death because the AB- at the blood bank had been exhausted and an alternative was needed urgently. Every second counts in this situation.

One of our colleagues who was a retired medical personnel asked if any of us had the Universal donor's status.

"What do you mean?" my husband asked

"Does anyone here have blood type O-? That's the universal donor's blood" he said.

"Oh I think Jonathan has that status" I grinned and answered. Immediately there was mild nervousness on Jonathan's face.

"Son it's time to save a life, we need around half a pint of blood to stabilize the patient," he said. Jonathan, mouth open and seeming lost in thought, after a few seconds, agreed to go on with the process.

The process was less than 10 minutes and Jonathan kept asking if the patient had been stabilized. Fortunately for us, the doctor came in with the news Jonathan craved.

"We'd like to say thank you Jonathan for your immense contribution towards saving the life of another. The world needs people with a heart like yours. The patient has been stabilized and hopefully, she'll recuperate seamlessly from now onward" The doctor said. Elated by the news from the doctor, Jonathan smiled like a baby that was tickled or given their favorite candy bar.

Throughout our journey back home, Jonathan smiles like the sun's rays. "You saved a life today son and I'm proud of you," my husband said to him. He felt fulfilled.

Blood type O- negative has been tagged one of the most important blood groups along with its positive counterpart in the world today because O- can donate to any other blood group without any complication, while O+ is the most popular blood type in the world. So maintaining a healthy diet that is specific to your blood type is equally as important as taking a shower every day.

Imagine if Jonathan had not taken care of himself with precise diet recommendations, he wouldn't have been in a better position to save the life of the young lady who needed an immediate transfusion from a healthy individual.

Mendel's Rule:

An Austrian scientist who lived in the 19th century, Gregor Mendel, was referred to as the "Father of Genetics" because of his incredible work and discoveries on inheritance. Several genetic patterns, principally controlled by the interactions between several allelcs, influence the inheritance of distinct blood types. The three primary alleles in the ABO blood group system are A, B, and O. An individual's blood type (A, B, AB, or O) is ultimately determined by these alleles that show which specific antigens are present on the surface of red blood cells or not. Alleles are unique gene variants with the same chromosomal location. You might ask what are Alleles? I'll try to explain it using cookbook terminology. So let's Imagine your genome(Genome is a full set of genetic information in an organism) as a cookbook like the one you reading. Each recipe represents a gene. One of the recipes is a banana pancake. Now let's imagine there's an updated edition of this cookbook most of which almost all the recipes are the same except for a few little brushes here and there like using a stainless pan or a non-stick pan to prepare your Banana Pancakes. Then a second edition of the cookbook came out, The Banana pancake recipe is still much present but now instead of only the pan changes, there is also a change in the variety of sugar used in the preparation of the Banana Pancake. So now you got three different alleles in the recipe of the Pancake, The first edition cookbook, the updated version, and then the second edition. Although they're all the same recipe, but because of the changes made in preparation methods, the final result will all taste different. DNA includes the instructions that determine a species's growth, how they function, and their physicalities. Different variants of a given trait can be produced by alleles, which differ in their DNA sequence.

For every gene, an individual receives two alleles, one from each parent. Alleles could be different as observed in this case or identical. In the latter case, they are designated as homozygous while the former are termed heterozygous. In essence, a person's genetic formulation is predicated on the combination of alleles he or she has inherited, which consequently affects the person's phenotype, i.e. his or her observable traits. It is the combination of these alleles which have been inherited from the two parents that determine whether a certain antigen will be present on the surface of red blood cells or not.Blood type A individuals express A antigens because they inherit one A allele and one O allele. Similar to this, people with blood type B express B antigens because they inherit one B allele and one O allele. Blood type O people do not express the A or B antigens and inherit two O alleles.

The Rh factor, which can be either positive or negative, is a significant antigen found in red blood cells in addition to the ABO blood group system. On the surface of red blood cells is a protein known as the Rh factor. You have Rh-positive blood cells if they contain this protein. You have Rh-negative blood if this protein is absent from your cells. An O-negative or positive blood type, for example, indicates your Rh status. The "positive" or "negative" parts of your blood refer to your Rh factor and varying diets can cause different kinds of reactions depending on whether it is present (rhesus positive) or absent(rhesus negative). Compared to rhesus-positive people, rhesus-negative people are more likely to develop immunoglobulin E allergies.

ABO and rhesus system correlations with some dietary parameters were found to be statistically significant; these correlations are also linked to certain diseases and their intermediate correlations with the blood system. While food preferences may not always be the direct cause of diseases, they can affect the risks associated with various diseases. So it is recommended blood type of an individual should be taken into consideration before any customized diet is made.

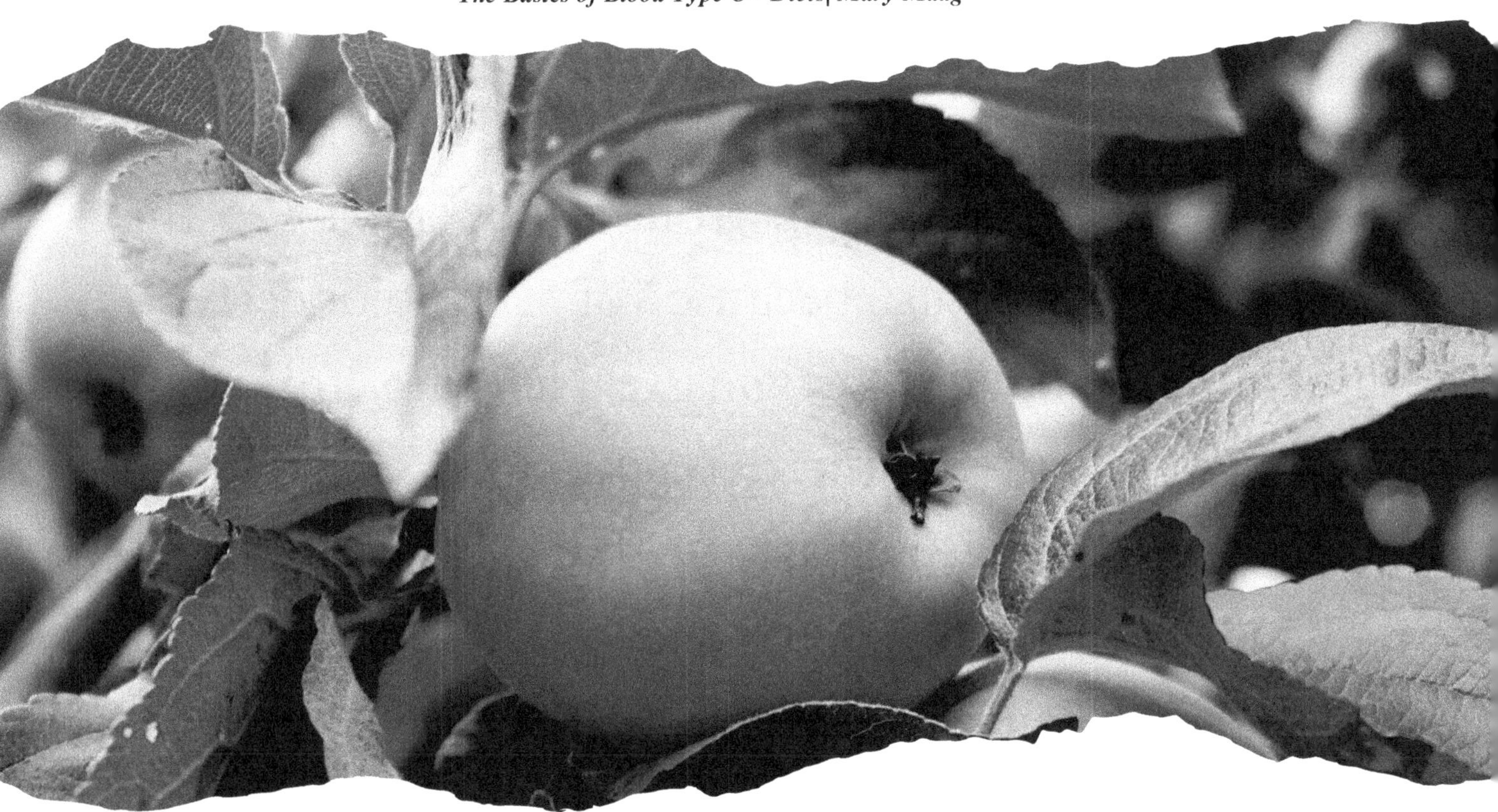

The Basics of Blood Type O- (negative) Diet

The fundamental principles of the blood type O-negative diet is that people with this distinct universal donor's blood may gain from following a diet specific to their genetic composition. Blood type O-negative diet expert practitioners recommend the following dietary guidelines:

Emphasis on Meat: Blood type O-negative proponents contend that individuals with this blood type may benefit from a diet similar to that of early humans because of the blood type's assumed ancestral origins, which are frequently linked to hunter-gatherer populations

Animal Protein Emphasis: People whose blood type is O-negative are also encouraged to prioritize animal proteins, particularly fish and lean meat.

Grain Reduction: Blood type O-negative diet may be recommended based on certain grains such as wheat and corn reduction or elimination. However, they might be more tolerant of some grains such as quinoa, rice, and oats. The ideology behind this is that some grains have a lower digestive compatibility with blood type O-negative people.

Eat Less Dairy: People with O-negative blood type are usually told to avoid consuming dairy products, particularly cow's milk. Instead, they can try using goat cheese, coconut milk, or almond milk as a substitute. The reason behind this is that the digestion systems of individuals with blood type O-negative can be incongruent or incompatible with dairy products, which may not be right for this type of relationship.

Fruits and Vegetables are Emphasized: Lots of fruits and vegetables, especially green ones like broccoli, spinach, and kale are recommended for people who have O-negative blood. This is because these foods are abundant in vitamins, minerals, and antioxidants which are important for general health and well-being.

The Focus is on Whole Foods: Processed or refined foods are generally avoided on the blood type O-nnegative diet. Rather, the stress is on whole unprocessed foods that come as close to nature as possible. This comprises healthy fats, nuts, seeds, fruits, vegetables, and lean proteins.

Mild Exercise: Although it has nothing to do with food, advocates of the blood type O-negative diet frequently stress the value of consistent exercise for those who have this blood type. Exercises like cardiovascular and strength training

Blood Type Connection

The Blood Type Diet was made popular by Dr. Peter D'Adamo, who suggested that a person's blood type have influences over how their body reacts to some food types. This notion argues that adhering to a diet that is blood type specific can better aid your digestion, enhance your immunity and foster smoother running of your body's internal mechanism.

Different blood types have different amounts of antigens and antibodies. Part of the Blood Type Diet is focused on lectins, a class of proteins. Cationic molecules can be bound to by lectins, a class of proteins with this property. Plant-based lectins also referred to as antinutrients, can cause nausea, vomiting, and flatulence in humans.

By customizing one's meals based on their unique blood group, they will increase the efficiency of the digestive system in breaking down food and avoid harmful effects associated with incompatible foods.

Type A blood types or the agrarian ones rely mainly on vegetables for nutrients. The blood type of the Nomads, type B, benefits greatly from a diet high in dairy products. For the Enigma blood type, Type AB, a combination of the Type A and Type B diets works best. Hunter blood type Type O, thought to be the oldest blood type, is best suited for a diet high in animal protein.

This book focuses on helping individuals with O-negative blood types develop diets that are tailored to them as they have certain features related to their kind of blood. 7% of people have an O-Negative blood type which is a universal donor. Persons who are Type O- negative often exhibit superior resistance to many fatal diseases due to various natural defences they possess.

The Importance of Eating According to Your Blood Type

The debate has been on for quite some time concerning eating for your blood type. Some argue that it is sometimes expensive to maintain a specific diet plan or routine. I say to people of such a nature to try being overweight, sick, or lose their good health. We all know that the cost of treating illnesses caused by bad dieting is far more expensive compared to eating specific diets professionally crafted for you, following expert advice so that your overall health improves exponentially.

So Just as no two fingerprints are alike, neither are the nutritional requirements of two people. A specially prepared meal aims to match dietary suggestions to your unique needs, taking into consideration other factors like age, gender, health issues, and, in the case of the Blood Type Diet, blood type. This special method aims to address unpleasant health issues as well as to increase your overall health and energy levels.

Personalized diet plans have advantages over generic ones, as evidenced by a growing body of research. Among the evidence in support are:

Improved Nutritional Intake: Studies showing that customized nutrition advice has a greater positive impact on food choices than general dietary guidelines were published in the Journal of Nutrition. By tailoring their diets, people can ensure they are getting the exact nutrients their bodies need.

Managing Allergies: According to the World Allergy Organization, specially prepared foods that exclude actual allergens reduce symptoms and improve the quality of life for those who suffer from food allergies.

Boosting Specific Health Conditions: Specific diet plans are highly beneficial for dealing with long term diseases. A study that was published a few years ago in Diabetes Care found that diabetic patients who had crafted special meal plans were able to achieve better blood sugar control than those who just followed the normal general guidelines.

Food Preferences: A study published in the Journal of Personalized Medicine found that diets specially prepared for an individual, have a higher chance that they will stick with it since they've developed the habit of choosing healthy foods.

Efficient Weight Loss: Contrary to standard diets, diet that was genetically customized resulted in more weight loss, according to a study that was published in the International Journal of Obesity.

Summary of Foods That Are Good for Blood Type O-negative

Most of the food we consume contains lectins, which are proteins expressed on the surface of red blood cells, and every blood group has a unique biochemistry. Therefore, it should come as no surprise that eating foods high in lectins that are incompatible with your blood type will interfere with hormonal homeostasis and digestion.

Cooking the right food based on your blood type is a masterful alternative to controlling your weight, lose weight, and maintain good health. Besides accomplishing your objective, unintended consequences or side effects are eliminated. The following is a list of foods that are generally thought to be good for people with blood type O-negative:

Lean Protein: It promotes rapid muscle regeneration and repair while supporting metabolic processes. Keep an eye on how much lean meat, fowl (particularly chicken and turkey), eggs, and lean beef or lamb cuts you consume.

Seafood: It's commonly recommended that those with blood type O-negative consume cold-water fish including halibut, mackerel, salmon, and cod. These fish are high in omega-3 fatty acids, which improve heart health and prevent inflammation.

Veggies: Eat mostly dark green vegetables like kale, spinach, and broccoli. Sweet potatoes, onions, garlic, and peppers are additional healthful vegetables for those who have blood type O-negative. Antioxidants, vitamins, and minerals are plenty in these veggies. Remember the more colored vegetables on your plate, the healthier it is.

Fruits: figs, plums, prunes, and berries should be eaten in moderation because moderation is key to many issues and they may be beneficial to blood type O-negative individuals because they contain antioxidants and other helpful nutrients.

Nuts: Try to eat nuts or use them to snack appropriately, with emphasis on almonds, walnuts, flaxseeds, and pumpkin seeds. They are rich in fiber, protein, and healthy fats, and these nuts and seeds can promote general health and well-being.

Good Fats: Include foods like avocado, and olive oil, and fatty fish like mackerel and salmon in your diet. These are good sources of fats. For people with blood type O-, these fats are thought to provide vital nutrients and support heart health.

Green Tea: They have a high antioxidant content and are thought to offer several health advantages, such as lowering inflammation and promoting metabolism.

Foods to Avoid or Limit

The great motivational speaker late Zig Ziglar said you shouldn't be a general wanderer but a meaningful specific, so why not make your diet also a meaningful specific? Blood Type O-negative diet hypothesis states that certain foods may not be optimal for people with this blood type. The O-negative person needs to know which foods to not consume or which he/she needs to stay away from to make good choices that will improve their health. The following is a list of foods that are usually suggested to be ditched when observing a Blood Type O-negative diet;

Dairy Products: People with blood type O–negative are generally advised against consuming dairy products, particularly those made from cow's milk. This covers ice cream, yogurt, cheese, and milk. Goat cheese, coconut milk, and almond milk are examples of substitutes that might be more tolerable for your system.

Grains: Avoid wheat and corn. Blood type O-negative might be able to tolerate grains like quinoa, rice, and oats better.

Legumes: Avoid consuming legumes, such as beans, lentils, and peanuts because you have less digestive compatibility with them.

Processed and Refined Foods: Avoid processed and refined foods like sugary snacks, white bread, and processed meats These foods may cause inflammation and create an internal body environment for diseases to thrive.

Fruits and Vegetables: Avoid or limit eggplants, tomatoes, and potatoes.

Oils: Avoid oils like peanuts, safflower, and corn oil. Instead use healthier alternatives like coconut oil, avocado oil, and olive oil.

Processed Meats: Avoid processed meats, including

sausage, bacon, and deli meats. These meats may include unhealthy additives and preservatives.

Highly Processed and Sugary Foods: Avoid highly processed and sugary foods, such as candies, sugary drinks, and desserts. These foods aggravate inflammation and causes other health problems.

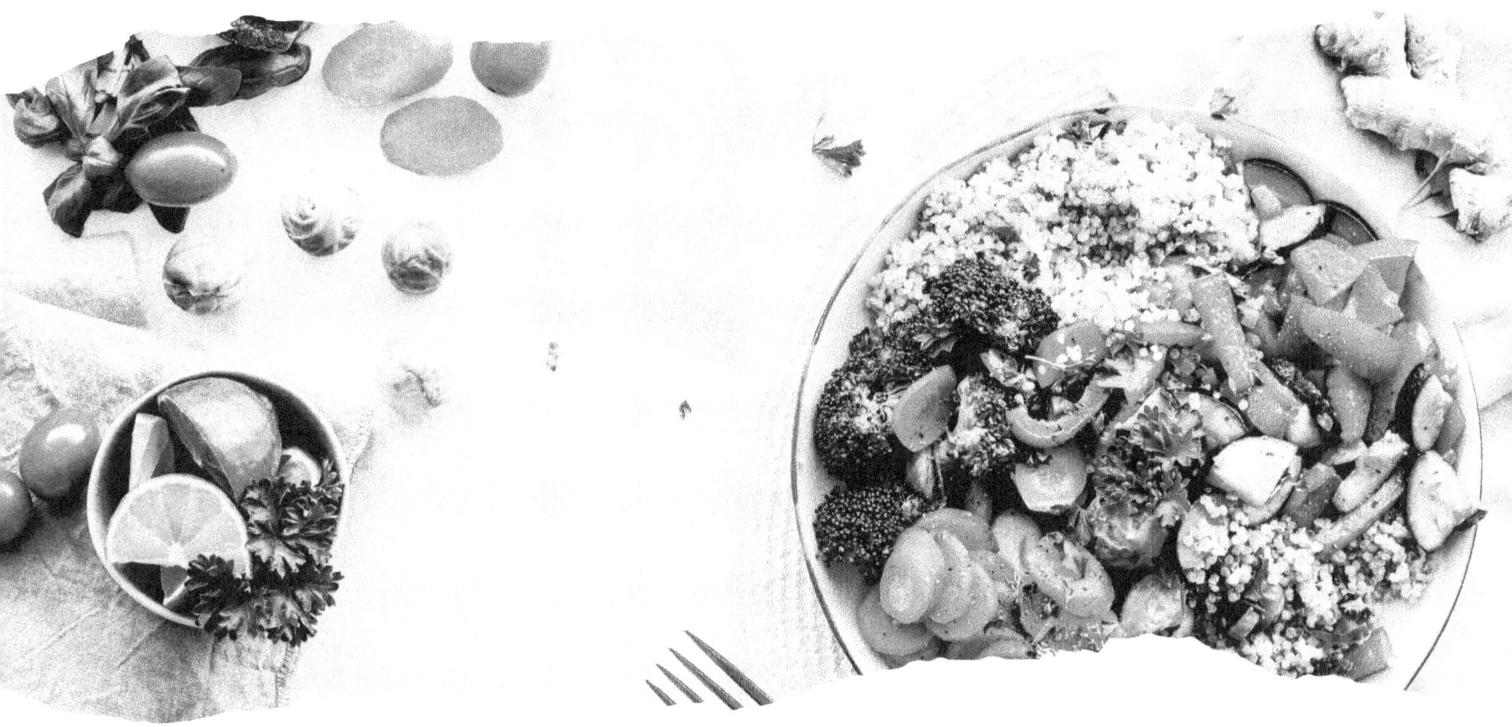

Nutritional Information

The nutritional information of every food is listed at the top of each outline. The calories, carbohydrates, fats, and protein are all listed in detail on the nutrition facts panel. Choosing the foods you need at a particular moment is made easier with the use of this data. When people are aware of the food they are consuming, they can carefully plan meals that will support their immediate health requirements.

People who want to make healthy food choices are empowered by this information provided.

Nutritional Profiles of Key Ingredients

The Blood Type O-negative diet is beneficial to health because it focuses on some specific nutrients. The following important nutrients are mostly highlighted for the Blood Type O-negative diet, although depending on the particular person:

Protein:

Lean meats and fish, poultry, eggs, lean lamb, and plant-based proteins like tempeh or tofu.

Iron:

Spinach, lean red meat, chicken, fish, beans, lentils, and fortified cereals.

Vitamin B12:

Plant-based foods like nutritional yeast, eggs, fish,

and cereals that are fortified.

Omega-3 Fatty Acids:
Walnuts, flaxseeds, fatty fish like salmon, mackerel,chia seeds, and sardines.

Vitamin D:

Fatty foods, eggs, and plant-based milks that have been fortified, as well as by spending time in the sun.

Antioxidants:

Berries, nuts, seeds, colorful fruits and vegetables, and herbs like ginger and turmeric.

Fiber:

fruits, vegetables, whole grains, beans, lentils, nuts, and seeds.

Calcium:

dairy products, almonds, tofu, leafy greens like collard greens and kale, and fortified plant-based milk.

Magnesium;

dark chocolate, whole grains, beans, nuts, and seeds, as well as leafy greens.

Water:

Water is necessary for maintaining digestion, transferring nutrients, removing toxins, and controlling body temperature.

Portion Sizes

Portion sizes are important for maintaining a healthy, balanced diet. Knowing how much or the quantity of what to eat not only supports mindful, intentional eating but also promotes overall well-being. Possessing the ability to understand portion sizes can help one's diet and overall health. A food that is rich in nutritional value can be used by a person through the practice of mindful eating and being conscious of the quantity as well as the quality of food eaten. Understanding portion sizes is crucial for optimizing nutrition. Further explanation includes:

1. Know your Calories: Portion sizes have a direct effect on the quantity of calories you eat. Portion excess could mean consuming too many calories and potentially gaining weight. Achieving calorie balance is crucial for weight management, and it can be done by paying attention to serving sizes.

2. Balanced Nutrient Distribution: Balanced nutrient distribution is likely guaranteed throughout the day with proper portion control. Meal portions should be appropriate so that different types of food can be included and a varied intake of vitamins and minerals is ensured.

3. Overeating: A person can accomplish eating less by using phases, portion size control which can help one to avoid overeating or gluttony. As a result of inner harmony and decreasing calories consumption, a lower chances of leading the life full of monotony and provides you with a balanced view to food.

4. Blood Sugar Regulation: One of the most effective ways for maintaining blood glucose levels stables is by controlling the quantities of what you consumed. Evenly spacing meals helps to control the amount of glucose released into the bloodstream which in turn doesn't shift the energy. It gives a steady supply of energy without crashes.

5. Individualization: Sizes of servings can be made appropriate to age of the person, the level of activity, and certain health goals.

7. Avoiding Nutrition Deficiencies: Keeping your food portion to the right amounts of nutritious components ensures you take sufficient of nutrients that your body needs. Going without binge food too much not only helps preserve your general health but also prevents essential nutrient deficiencies. However, adding diet supplement can be a solution in this situation as well.

8. Weight Control: In fact, one of the key aspects of staying fit and healthy is a developed portion control plan. Incorporation of planned portions in the diet proves to be a better way to not only be deliberate but also efficient, the benefit of which can be realized for both the outcomes of weight loss, maintenance, and gain whichever the case might be.

Tips for Portion Control

- **Use Visual Cues:** You should familiarize yourself with visual cues in terms of portion size such as using your hands to measure grains, veggies, and proteins.

- **Go through the package correctly and read food labels,** to determine calories and serving sizes. Considering each package's servings count contributes to avoiding excess food intake.

- **Recognize Your Hunger Cues:** Don't get distracted from your own true goal: keep your mind awake and attentive. Consume food in moderation. Know when your tummy is filled up already.

- **Plate Composition:** Aim to get half of your meal comprised of whole grains, a block of lean protein, and veggies. This then ensures that balanced meals that are eye-catchy are offered.

The Importance of Balanced Nutrition

Nutrition that incorporates a wide range of foods in suitable amounts is fundamental to overall health and wellness. It requires eating diverse foods in right proportions to give the body the essential nutrients it requires to work optimally. Below are the key reasons why attaining and keeping balanced nutrition is vital:

1.**Consumption of Vital Minerals:** So a balanced diet to the body consists of a proportionate amount of protein, fats, carbs, and other nutrients it needs. This nutrient is for the body an important fuel for the different vital functions it performs like growth, development, and the maintenance of good health.Energy-producing macronutrients for the body are proteins, lipids, and carbohydrates. To support daily activities, work, exercise, and general vitality, a balanced diet ensures that energy requirements are met.

2. **Controlling Weight**: The needed weigh is maintained by a balanced diet. By consuming a varied diet of plentiful nutrient-rich food, along with proper portion sizes, individuals are able to obtain and maintain a healthy body weight.

3. **Enhanced Emotion and Mental Well-Being:** Found in various foods and notably prominent in fishes, omega-3 fatty acids have been linked to mental wellness and good mood. Vitamins B6 and B12 are the other nutrients that are related to improved mental health. Consumption of a balanced diet helps isolate the risk factors of a huge number of mental disorders and has a positive impact on mental health.

4. **Regulation of Blood Sugar:** Dietary composition which includes carbohydrates, proteins, vitamins, and minerals supports maintaining blood sugar levels. The selection of complex carbohydrates with proteins and fats can help to keep a steady blood

sugar, this will help to block spikes and crashes of the blood sugar that occur throughout the day.

5. **Optimal Digestive Health:** A diet abundant in fiber, obtained from fruits, vegetables, and whole grains, promotes healthy digestion and regular bowel movements. Fiber also contributes to a feeling of fullness, supporting weight management.

6. **Healthy Bones:** Calcium and vitamin D intake in green leafy foods, dairy, and sunlight are some healing agents for stronger bones. This gives people a chance to grow stronger and as a result, prevent osteoporosis and other ailments.

9. **Hormonal Balance:** Nutrient-dense foods contribute to hormonal balance, supporting reproductive health, metabolism, and overall hormonal function. This is especially important for women's health.

This page intentionally left blank

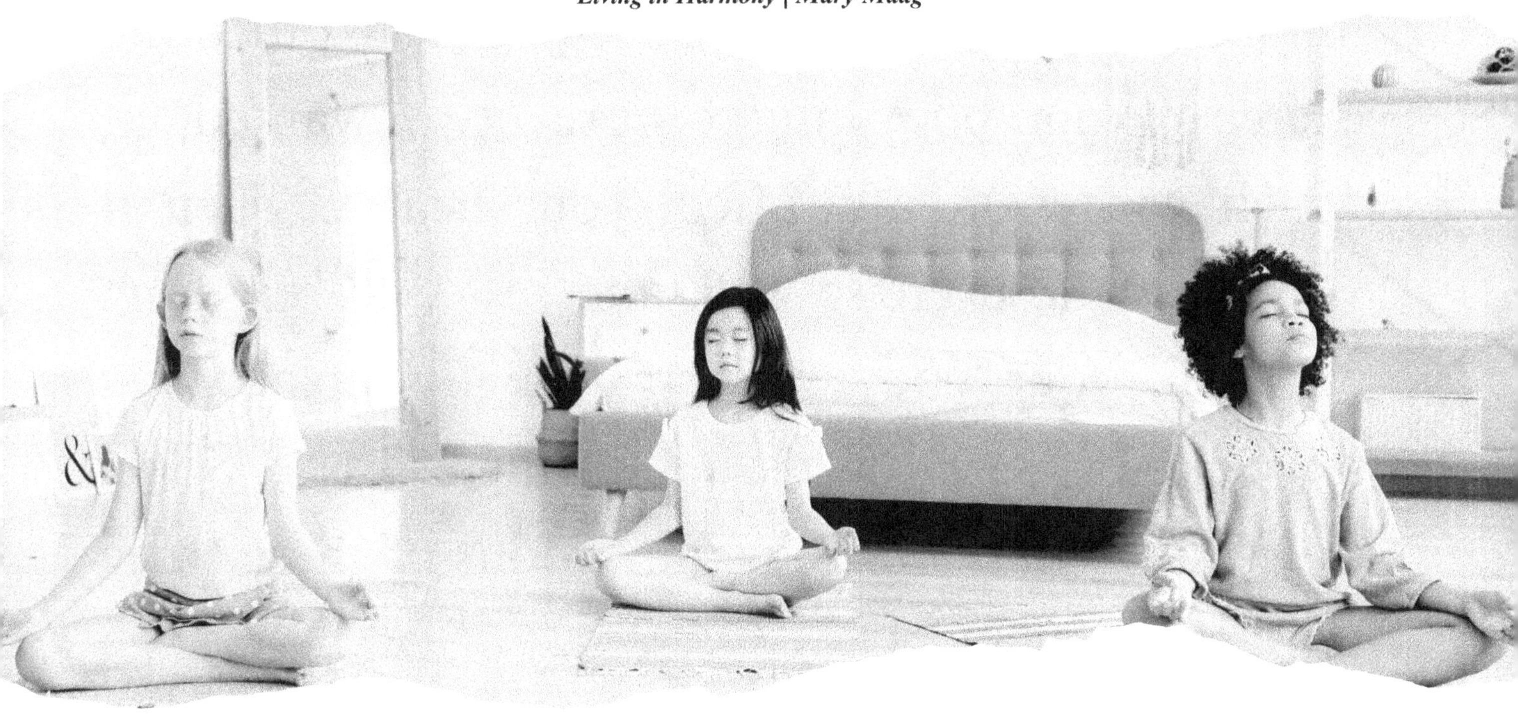

LIVING IN HEALTHY HARRMONY

Achieving optimal health for people with Blood Type O- negative goes beyond just diet. It is important as a human being to incorporate both regular exercise and enough rest into your lifestyle for absolute well-being. Diet, Exercise, and Rest are correlated in that when one is neglected, it tends to affect the others. If you eat well, and exercise well but don't rest well, your result will be minimal. If you eat well, and rest well but don't exercise, your body might store up unwanted fat which will eventually affect your health. Then if you're able to exercise well, and rest well but don't eat well, your body will struggle to replace lost nutrients or worn-out tissues during exercise. Some of the advantages of the connections of these three musketeers include:

1. Exercise Helps Enhance how the Blood Type O-negative Diet works:

Exercising helps by promoting the weight management of the person and then optimizing their metabolic function. Physical activities improve the body's ability to utilize various nutrients smoothly, working systematically with the dietary guidelines for Blood Type O-negative.

2. Certain Exercises benefits Blood Type O-negative people:

Aerobic, strength tr, and agility-based activities like sprinting or martial arts align well with the good nature of a blood type O-negative person.

3. Resting enough Allows the Body to Recover and Repair itself.

Enough rest is very important in the wellness equation for Blood Type O- negative people as well as the other blood group members. Restful periods optimize the body's ability to recover and repair itself, enhancing the benefits of both exercise and a special diet.

4. Balancing of Exercise Intensity and Duration.

Blood Type O-negative people need to know that the exact intensity they need when working out should vary as also the time they have to spend on a particular session or station. While their nature may permit intense workouts, adequate recovery time is crucial to prevent training too much with less time for recovery.

5. Circadian Rhythms and Sleep Quality

People with Blood Type O-negative might gain from planning their workouts around their bodies' normal daily
cycles. Circadian rhyme is our body's internal clock. You should prioritize getting a good sleep at night after the day's tedious work.

6. Stress Management.

Managing stress levels is very important to your health, as chronic stress can have dangerous effects on you leading to various problems like insomia, hypertension, etc. Blood type O-negative people may benefit from adding stress-relieving techniques such as yoga or meditation to their daily routine lifestyle.

7. Consulting Health Experts.

It is recommended that individuals with Blood Type O+ speak with medical professionals or fitness experts before beginning a new exercise program, particularly if they have pre-existing medical conditions. This guarantees that the fitness regimen is customized to meet the requirements of each person and take their health into account.

Exercise Choices for Blood Type O-negative Individuals

Physical activity that corresponds with the unique characteristics and evolutionary history of people with Blood Type O-negative can enhance their general well-being. However, different likes and abilities exist among people making some forms of physical activity to be commonly viewed as more advantageous for someone with the blood type O-negative. The following exercise categories may be beneficial to people with blood type O-negative :

1. Aerobic exercises: Some examples are cycling, swimming, jogging, and brisk walking.

Reason: This aerobic exercise helps in maintaining a healthy heart and efficient blood circulation. Such cardiovascular exercises maintain the strong heart and robust metabolism inherent in Blood Type O-negative individuals.

2. High-Intensity Interval Training (HIIT): These include such exercises as intervals, circuit training, and sprints.

Reason: HIIT is best suited for Blood Type O's dynamic high-energy personality. Short bursts of intense exercise interspersed with rest meet their need for diverse hard workouts.

3. Strength training activities such as bodyweight exercises, resistance training, weightlifting

Reason: Muscle mass has to be maintained or even built up by those who are Blood Type O-negative . In addition to promoting physical resilience, strength training enhances bone health and metabolic efficiency.

4. Martial Arts: Brazilian Jiu-Jitsu, Kung Fu, Taekwondo, and Karate.

Blood Type O-negative is among the most rare blood type in the world with only 7% of people having this blood. People who have this type of blood are found to be agile and adaptable by nature just like some martial artists since these activities involve mental concentration combined with physical flexibility and strength.

5. Team Sports: Rugby, basketball, and football among others.

Therefore, individuals with Blood Type O- negative

frequently perform well in social and collaborative environments. Besides just physical fitness, engaging in team sports also fosters unity and camaraderie.

6. Agility Exercises: Dance, obstacle courses and agility drills among other options.

So one may want to consider agility and coordination exercises as good for those with Blood Type O-negative. Also, these activities can enhance general physical ability; they're dynamic just like their counterparts are.

7. Outdoor Activities: Running trails, rock climbing or going on hikes

Accordingly, whenever people with Blood Type O engage in outdoor activities that bring them closer to nature their innate instincts are heightened leading to a sense of renewal both physically and mentally. These pursuits will allow you renew your body as well as mind.

8. Mind-Body Exercises: Pilates yoga etc.

However, mindfulness techniques such as yoga can help balance this preference since people with blood type 'O' tend to enjoy dynamic actions more than any other practice that requires calmness. Yoga including pilates helps improve core strength , flexibility & enhances mental health.

9. Diverse, Frequent Exercise:

Reason: To avoid boredom and raise general fitness levels, people with blood type O may benefit from a variety of exercises. A well-rounded regimen is ensured by including cardio, strength training, and flexibility. The best workout regimen matches personal preferences, degree of fitness, and health-related variables. A sustainable, pleasurable fitness journey is facilitated by tailoring workouts and paying attention to your body.

The Role of Good Rest In Ultimate Health

Rest is a fundamental part of life and the amount of rest you need depends on you as an individual and how rigorous your daily activities are. Rest plays a vital role in maintaining our body's state of emotional, psychological, and physical health. In our digital world today, getting enough sleep is very important for maintaining good health and well-being. Sleep helps our body to recharge and repair damaged cells effectively and also gives the immune system the right space to carry out their rigorous activities. The following ideas may assist you in obtaining the restorative sleep that your body and mind require:

1. Make Effort to Maintain a Regular Sleep Schedule:

The body's internal clock is known as the circadian rhythm. If a person maintain a regular sleep schedule, their body can function at its peak and prepare itself for the necessary repairs and brain clearing that take place while they sleep.

2. Set or create a Bedtime Routines

For your body to recognize that it is almost time for bed consistently, a habit needs to be created around your routine or bedtime rituals. Rituals like light stretching, meditation, reading a book, drinking green tea, listening to relaxing music, or cold shower.

3. Limit your screen time before bed:

The blue light from your phones, tablets, and computer screens can interfere with the production of melatonin, so avoid using any of your digital gadgets
at least an hour before bed.

4. Eat your Dinners Earlier:

If you have to have dinner, do that at least 3 hours before bed. Stay away from large meals, coffee, and too much liquids right before bed.

5. Engage in Daytime Exercise:

Frequent exercise during the day enhances sleep, the vitamin D you get from the sun also helps you sleep well. However, vigorous exercise right before bed can be disruptive.

6. Don't Take Midday Naps:

To preserve the quality of your nighttime sleep, napping should be limited to 20 to 30 minutes and avoided right before bed.

7. Choose a Comfortable Sleep Position:

Try out different sleeping positions, pillows, and mattresses to see what aligns and comforts your body properly.

8. Stay away from from Stimulants:

Steer clear of stimulants like caffeine, nicotine, and other substances during the evening and night.

9. Schedule Relaxation Time Before Sleep

Before going to bed, spend an hour reading, having a warm bath, or engaging in other soothing activities.nAssess and Modify Your Bedroom Setting , Examine your bedroom for problems with light, noise, or your mattress and adjust as necessary to create the ideal sleeping environment.

This page intentionally left blank

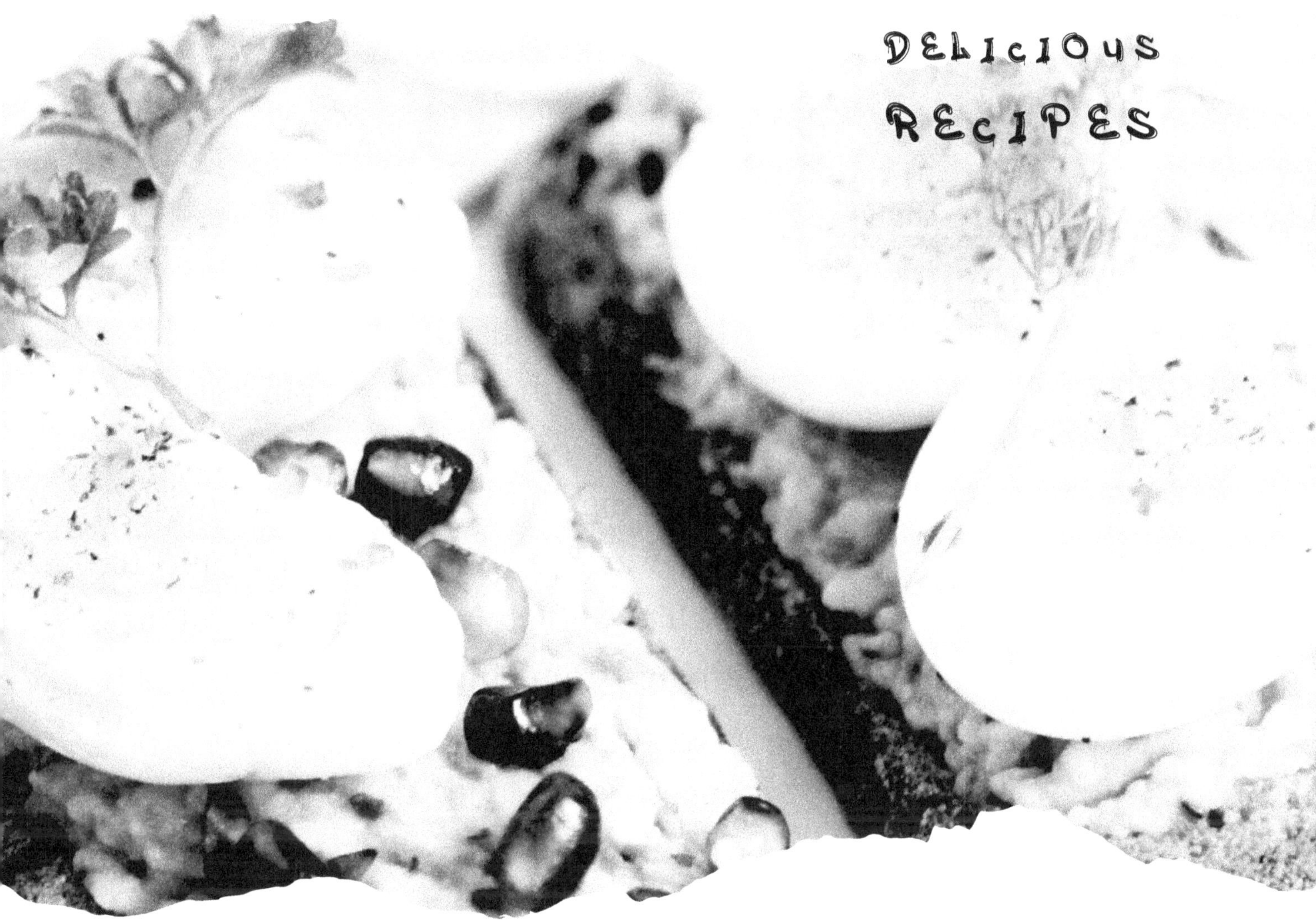

BREAKFAST RECIPES

FOR HEALTHY YOU

Scrambled Eggs with Zucchini

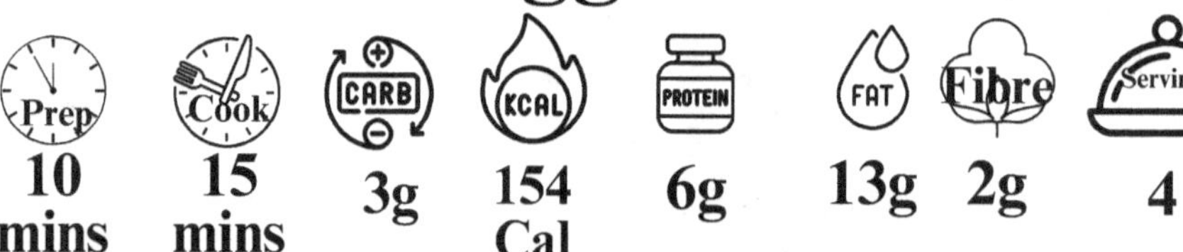

Prep	**Cook**	**CARB**	**KCAL**	**PROTEIN**	**FAT**	**Fibre**	**Servings**
10 mins	**15 mins**	**3g**	**154 Cal**	**6g**	**13g**	**2g**	**4**

Ingredients

- 4 large eggs, lightly beaten
- 2 Tsp grated Parmesan cheese
- 2 Tsp olive oil
- 1 zucchini, sliced 1/8- to 1/4-inch thick
- 1/4 Tsp garlic powder, or to taste
- salt and ground black pepper to taste

Instructions

1.In a larger dish, stir together beaten eggs and Parmesan cheese; put aside.

2. In a big skillet set over medium-high heat, warm up the olive oil. Sauté the zucchini in high oil for about 7 minutes, turning from time to time, or until softened and gently browned. Add pepper, salt, and garlic powder for seasoning.

3. Lower the heat to medium and cover the zucchini in the skillet with the egg mixture. Stir gently and cook for approximately 3 minutes. After turning off the heat, place a lid on the skillet and wait another two minutes or more, or until the eggs are set..

MY OBSERVATIONS

Omelette with Vegetables

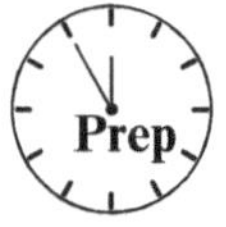  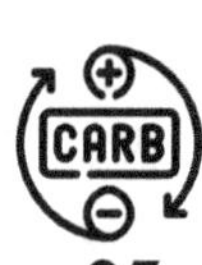  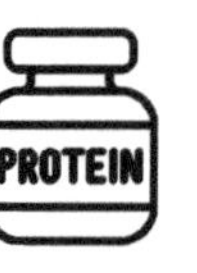 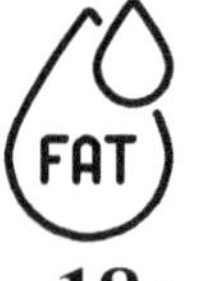 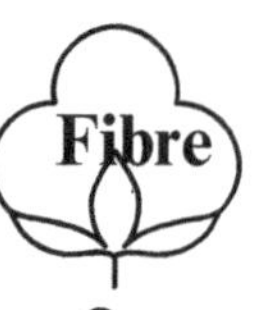 

Prep	Cook	CARB	KCAL	PROTEIN	FAT	Fibre	Servings
10 mins	10 mins	25g	141 Cal	7g	18g	2g	2

Ingredients

- 2 Tsp butter, divided
- 1 small onion, chopped
- 1 green bell pepper, chopped
- ¾ Tsp salt, divided
- 4 large eggs
- 2 Tsp milk
- ⅛ Tsp freshly ground black pepper
- 2 ounces shredded Swiss cheese

Instructions

1.Melt 1 tablespoon butter in a medium skillet over medium heat. Cook and stir onion and bell pepper in butter until just tender, 4 to 5 minutes. Transfer vegetables to a bowl, season with 1/4 teaspoon salt, and set aside.

2.Beat together eggs, milk, remaining 1/2 teaspoon salt, and pepper in a separate bowl.

3.In the skillet over medium heat, melt the remaining tablespoon of butter and swirl to coat the skillet bottom with butter. Pour in egg mixture and heat, stirring occasionally, until bottoms of eggs start to set, about 1 minute, after butter has melted. Using a spatula, gently lift the omelet's edges so that any egg that isn't cooked can spill onto the skillet. Cook for an additional one to two minutes, or until the middle of the omelet begins to look dry.

4.Drizzle the omelet with cheese, then cover half of it with the veggie mixture. Gently fold omelet over vegetables with spatula. Simmer for about a minute, or until cheese melts to the desired consistency. Transfer the omelet to a dish. After cutting in half, serve.

MY OBSERVATIONS

Smoked Salmon and Avocado Toast

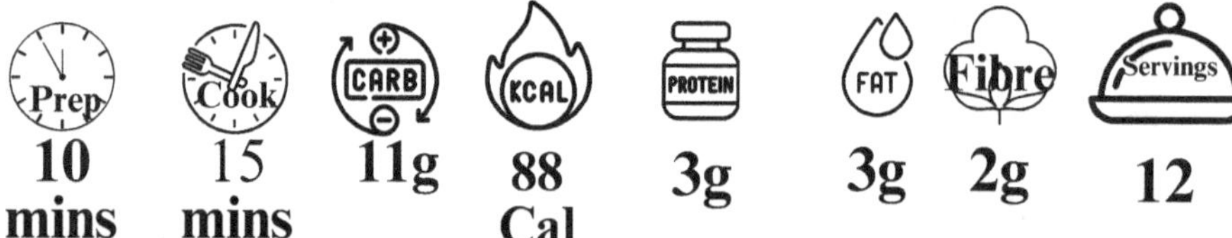

Prep	Cook	CARB	KCAL	PROTEIN	FAT	Fibre	Servings
10 mins	15 mins	11g	88 Cal	3g	3g	2g	12

Ingredients

- 1 ripe avocado, pitted
- 2 Tsp lemon juice
- 1 Tsp minced fresh tarragon
- 24 toasted cocktail-size slices pumpernickel bread or melba toasts
- 2 ounces smoked salmon, cut into 24 pieces
- 1 Tsp coarse Maldon sea salt
- Fresh tarragon sprigs, capers, sliced cornichons or olives, poppy or sesame seeds, lemon zest and/or red onion for garnish

Instructions

1.In a bowl, mash avocado with tarragon and lemon juice. Distribute around one teaspoon of the mixture onto every slice of toast or bread. Place salmon on top and season with salt. As desired, garnish.

MY OBSERVATIONS

Quinoa Breakfast Bowl

  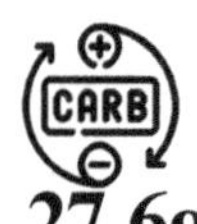  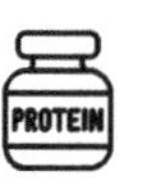 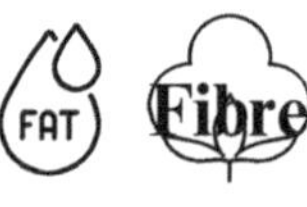 

Prep	Cook	CARB	KCAL	PROTEIN	FAT	Fibre	Servings
5 mins	20 mins	27.6g	232 Cal	5.7g	11.5g	3.3g	4

Ingredients

- 3/4 cup dry quinoa
- 1 1/2 cups water
- 3/4 cup canned coconut milk
- 1/2 cup non-dairy milk, plus more for topping
- 1 date, chopped, or 1 Tsp maple syrup (optional)
- 2 Tsp ground cinnamon
- 2 Tsp vanilla extract
- Pinch of salt
- Toppings for you! (banana, coconut flakes, walnuts, chia seeds, chocolate chips)

Instructions

1.Combine water and quinoa in a medium-sized pot. Bring to a boil, then lower the heat to a simmer, cover, and cook until the quinoa is frothy, 13 to 15 minutes. Maintain a low heat setting.

2.Add salt, sweetener, cinnamon, vanilla, and coconut or nondairy milk. Mix everything together. Cook until the quinoa is still pourable but has absorbed most of the milk. If more nondairy milk is required, add it.

3.Transfer some into a dish and garnish with additional nondairy milk and your preferred toppings, such as fruit, almonds, or nuts—the options are unlimited!

MY OBSERVATIONS

Spinach and Mushroom Frittata

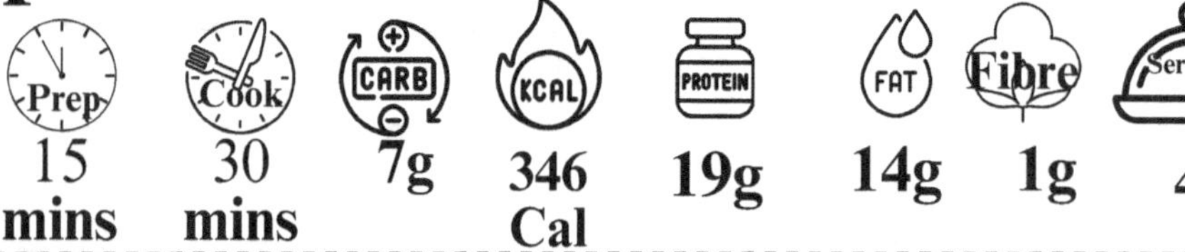

Prep	Cook	CARB	KCAL	PROTEIN	FAT	Fibre	Servings
15 mins	30 mins	7g	346 Cal	19g	14g	1g	4

Ingredients

- 6 eggs
- 1/4 cup (60 ml) milk
- 1 cup (250 ml) grated cheddar cheese
- 1 onion, thinly sliced
- 4 oz (115 g) white button mushrooms, sliced
- 3 Tsp (45 ml) butter
- 2 cups (500 ml) baby spinach
- Salt and pepper

Instructions

1. Oven temperature should be set to 180 °C (350 °F) with the rack in the middle position. Grease a baking dish that is 20 cm (8 inches) square. Put away. Whisk the eggs and milk together in a large bowl. Add the cheese. Add little pepper and salt for seasoning. Set bowl aside. Melt butter in a large nonstick skillet and cook the onion and mushrooms over medium heat. Add little pepper and salt for seasoning.

2. Stirring frequently, sauté the spinach for about a minute after adding it. Transfer the mushroom mixture to the egg mixture.

3. Mix thoroughly and transfer into a baking dish. Bake for about twenty-five minutes, or until the frittata is puffy and gently browned. With a spatula, divide the frittata into four squares and take it out of the plate. It's ready to be served warm when you place it on a platter.

74

MY OBSERVATIONS

Brown Rice Pancake

 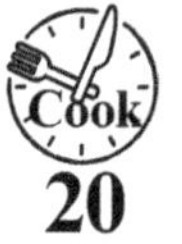 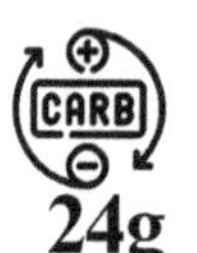  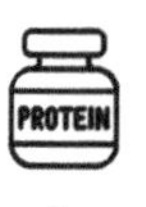 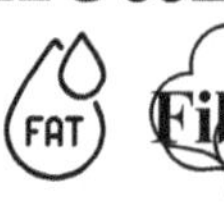 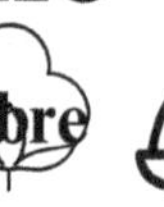 

Prep	Cook	CARB	KCAL	PROTEIN	FAT	Fibre	Servings
5 mins	20 mins	24g	159 Cal	4g	5g	1g	6

Ingredients

- 1 cup of flour made from brown rice
- One-third cup sugar and one-quarter teaspoon of gluten-free double-acting baking powder
- A smidgeon of kosher salt
- 2 eggs
- Half a cup of whole milk
- 1 tsp of vegetable oil
- 1 tsp vanilla essence

Instructions

1. Whisk the eggs, milk, oil, and vanilla extract in a sizable mixing basin.
2. Mix in the sea salt, sugar, baking powder, and brown rice flour until no big clumps remain.
3. Heat up some oil in a nonstick skillet or pan over medium-high heat.
4. When the pan is hot, transfer batter into it with a ladle or ¼ measuring cup.
5. After about three minutes, or until air bubbles begin to form on the surface of the pancake, flip it.
6. Simmer for a further one to two minutes. Test the doneness of the pancake by poking it lightly in the centre; if it comes out firm, it's done.
7. Serve hot with maple syrup and fruit toppings.

MY OBSERVATIONS

Cherry Scones

  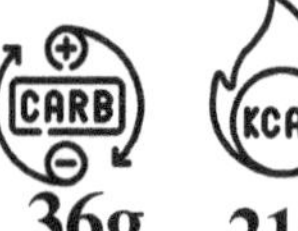 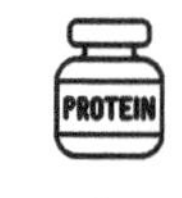 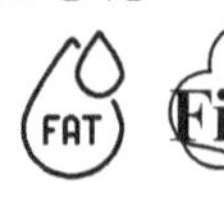 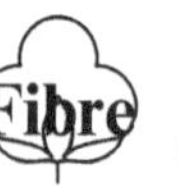 

Prep	Cook	CARB	KCAL	PROTEIN	FAT	Fibre	Servings
10 mins	19 mins	36g	218 Cal	4g	8g	1g	12

Ingredients

- 2 ½ Cups (313 grams) All Purpose Flour
- ⅓ Cup (67 grams) Granulated Sugar
- 1 Tsp Baking Powder
- 2 Tsp Lemon Zest
- 2 Tsp Orange Zest
- ½ Tsp Kosher Salt
- 6 Tsp Unsalted Butter
- ½ Cup (125 ml) Heavy Whipping Cream
- 1 Tsp Vanilla Extract
- 1 Tsp Almond Extract
- 1 Large Egg
- 1 Large Egg Yolk
- 1 ½ Cups Bing Cherries pitted, cut into quarters

Instructions

1. Adjust the oven temperature to 425 F (218 C) and place parchment paper on a baking pan.
2. Mix the flour, sugar, baking powder, orange and lemon zests, and salt in a medium-sized bowl.
3. Using a pastry grinder or your fingers, cut in the cold butter cubes until they resemble cornmeal.
4. For ten minutes, place the flour mixture in the freezer.
5. Whisk together the egg, egg yolk, cream, almond extract, and vanilla extract in a another basin.
6. Take the flour mixture out of the freezer and add the cream and egg combination. Using a wooden spoon, stir until just combined, then loosely shape into a ball with your hands.
7. Knead dough with chopped cherries on a floured surface.
8. Approximately 2 inches thick, form into a circle. After cutting the circle in half, divide each half into thirds(6trian)

78

9. Scones should be spaced 1.5–2 inches apart on a baking sheet.

10. Apply a thin layer to the scones using the three tablespoons of heavy cream that are left, or more if necessary.

11. Bake for 18 to 20 minutes, until the edges are brown.

12. Wait ten minutes for the pan to cool on the oven rack before removing the scones and serving!

MY OBSERVATIONS

Broccoli Feta Frittata

 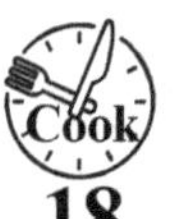 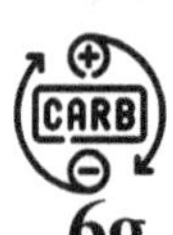  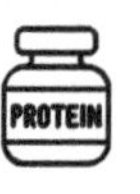 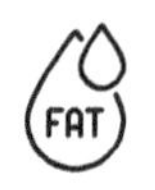 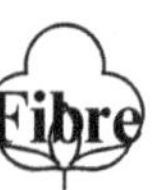 

Prep	Cook	CARB	KCAL	PROTEIN	FAT	Fibre	Servings
5 mins	18 mins	6g	232 Cal	16g	8g	1g	4

Ingredients

- 1 tsp unsalted butter
- ½ onion, finely diced
- 2 cups chopped broccoli florets
- Salt and pepper
- 7 large eggs
- 3 ounces feta, crumbled

Instructions

1. Melt butter over medium heat in an 8-inch ovenproof nonstick skillet or seasoned cast-iron pan. Add onion and simmer for about 4 minutes, stirring now and again, until transparent. Add the broccoli, season with salt and pepper, and simmer for a further six minutes or until it is just cooked, stirring from time to time.

2. Adjust an oven rack to be 4 inches from the heat source and preheat the broiler to high. Add more pepper and salt to the eggs as you beat them together in a medium-sized bowl. Drizzle eggs over onion-broccoli mixture, toss to incorporate, then sprinkle feta on top. Cook for about five minutes, without stirring, or until eggs are set through on the bottom and starting to set on top.

3. Place the pan in the oven and broil for two to three minutes, or until the eggs are set and starting to brown. Slice into wedges and proceed to serve.

MY OBSERVATIONS

Pear Rosemary Bread

  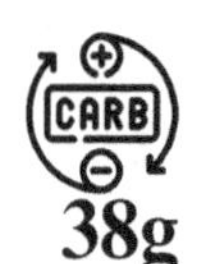 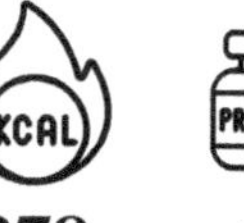 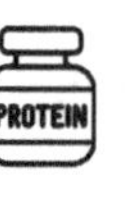 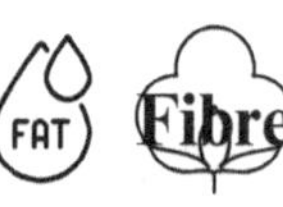 

Prep	Cook	CARB	KCAL	PROTEIN	FAT	Fibre	Servings
15 mins	90 mins	38g	278 Cal	4g	14g	2g	20

Ingredients

- 3 cups all-purpose flour
- 1 tsp ground cinnamon
- 1 tsp salt
- 1 teaspoon baking soda
- ¼ tsp baking powder
- 2 cups white sugar
- 2 cups peeled shredded pears
- 1 cup chopped pecans
- 3 large eggs
- ¾ cup vegetable oil
- 2 tsp vanilla extract.

Instructions

1. Set the oven's temperature to 325°F, or 165°C. Grease and flour two 8 by 5-inch loaf pans lightly.

2. In a large mixing basin, combine flour, baking powder, baking soda, cinnamon, and salt; create a well in the center.

3. In a separate bowl, thoroughly incorporate the grated pears, sugar, pecans, eggs, oil, and vanilla. Pour the mixture into the dry ingredients well and stir until it is barely moistened. Fill loaf pans with batter using a spoon.

4. Bake for one hour and fifteen minutes in a preheated oven. Before removing from the loaf pans, let cool on a wire rack.

MY OBSERVATIONS

Maple Sausage Scramble

  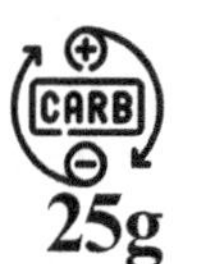 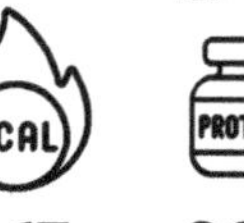 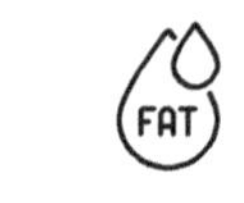 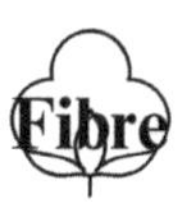 

Prep	Cook	CARB	KCAL	PROTEIN	FAT	Fibre	Servings
10 mins	14 mins	25g	467 Cal	22g	31g	2g	4

Ingredients

- 1 Tbsp. Olive Oil
- 1/2 Package Four Brothers® Smoked Maple Sausage, coarsely chopped
- 2 C. Frozen Potatoes O'Brien
- 1 Tsp Maple Syrup
- 8 Large Eggs
- 3 Green Onions, thinly sliced plus additional for serving (optional)
- 1/4 tsp. Kosher Salt
- 1/4 tsp. Ground Black Pepper
- Hot Sauce for Serving (optional)

Instructions

1. Set the flat-top grill outside to medium heat. Oil the grill. Stir regularly and simmer for 8 minutes, or until the sausage and potatoes are lightly browned. Add the syrup, and heat for one minute, or until browned.

2. Whisk eggs, onions, salt, and pepper in a medium-sized basin. Scramble the egg mixture and add it to the sausage mixture on the grill. Cook for 4 minutes, or until the desired doneness, stirring now and again. Yields approximately six cups.

3. If preferred, top the scramble with spicy sauce and onions.

MY OBSERVATIONS

This page was intentionally left blank.

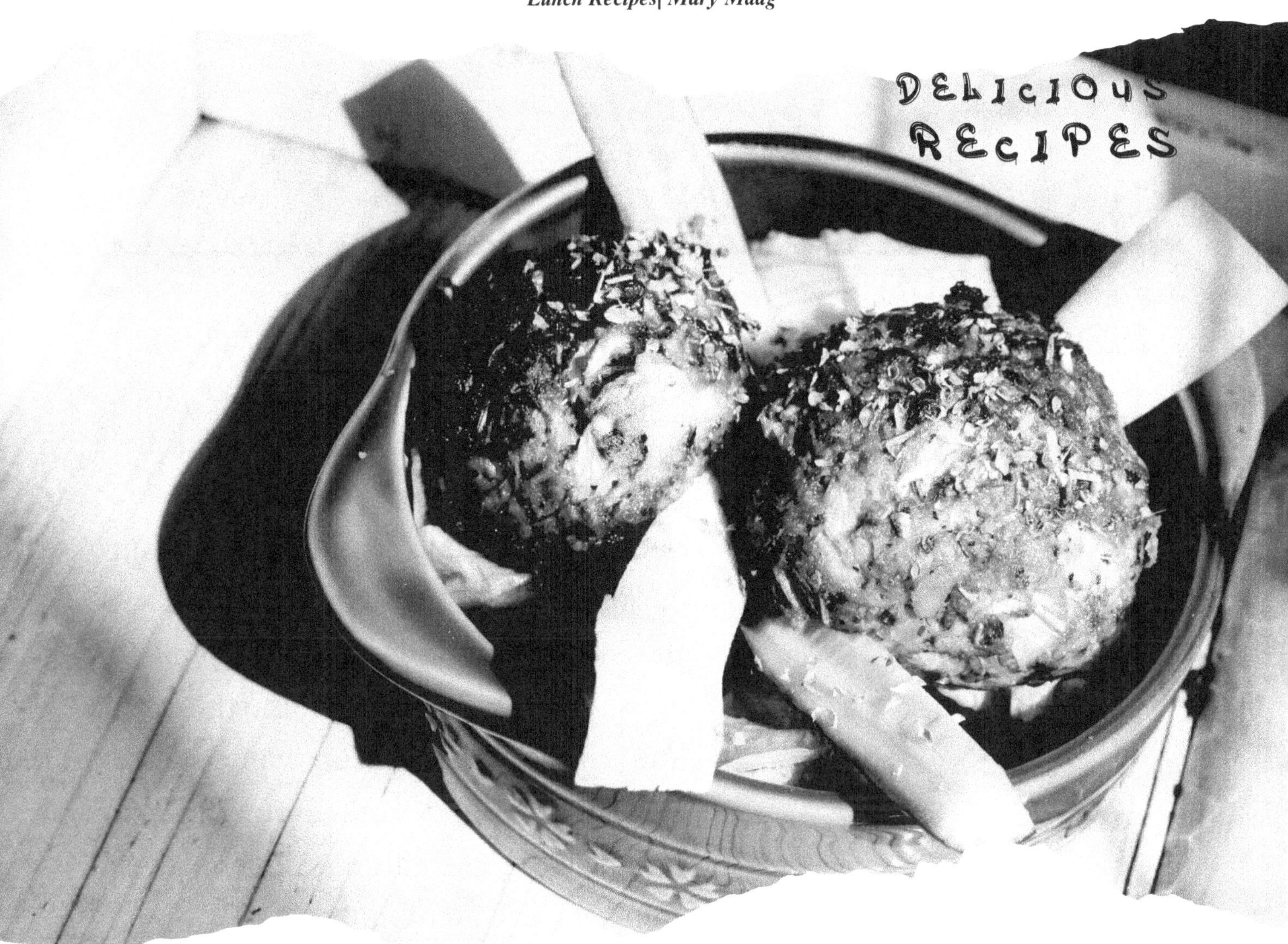

LUNCH
RECIPES

—— FOR HEALTHY YOU ——

Baked Falafel

  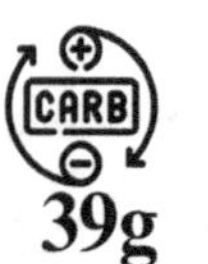 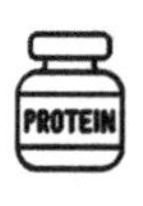 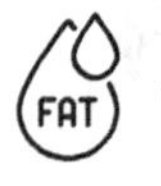 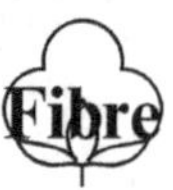 

Prep	Cook	CARB	KCAL	PROTEIN	FAT	Fibre	Servings
20 mins	25 mins	39g	281 Cal	11g	9g	7g	2

Ingredients

- 1/4 cup finely chopped onion
- Rinse and drain one fifteen-ounce can of garbanzo beans.
- 1/2 cup freshly chopped parsley
- minced three garlic cloves
- One tsp of ground cumin
- 1/2 tsp of coriander powder
- Half a tsp of salt
- Half a tsp of baking soda
- 1 spoonful of flour for all purposes
- 1 beaten egg
- 2 tsp olive oil

Instructions

1. After wrapping the onion in cheesecloth, try to extract as much moisture as you can. Put aside. In a food processor, combine the garbanzo beans, parsley, garlic, cumin, coriander, salt, and baking soda. Blend the contents until a coarse purée is achieved. In a bowl, combine the onion and the garbanzo bean combination. Add the egg and flour and stir. Form into four sizable patties and let aside to stand for fifteen minutes.

2. Heat the oven to 400 degrees Fahrenheit, or 200 degrees Celsius.

3. In a large ovenproof skillet, heat the olive oil over medium-high heat. After adding the patties to the skillet, fry for 3 minutes on each side, or until golden brown.

4. After moving the skillet to the oven, preheat it for about ten minutes, or until it is thoroughly heated.

MY OBSERVATIONS

Lamb meatball

  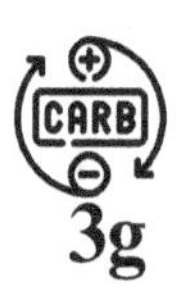 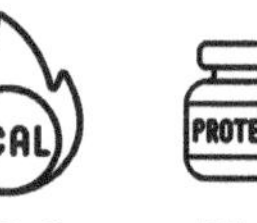 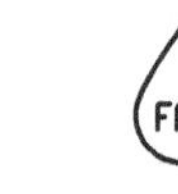 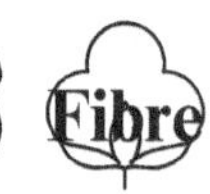 

Prep	Cook	CARB	KCAL	PROTEIN	FAT	Fibre	Servings
25 mins	30 mins	3g	136 Cal	7g	10g	0.1g	24

Ingredients

- 1 tsp of butter without salt
- 5finely chopped shallots
- 2 pounds of lamb, ground
- 1 cup of bread crumbs
- ¼ cup of freshly chopped parsley
- 1 egg, whisked
- two tsp lemon zest
- One-half tsp dried marjoram
- To taste, add salt and freshly ground black pepper.
- ½ cup butter without salt
- One tsp of olive oil
- 2 ½ tsp of tomato sauce
- Half a cup of wine
- 1 little clove of chopped garlic
- One dab of ground cinnamon

Instructions

1. One tablespoon of butter should be melted over medium heat in a skillet. Add the shallots to the skillet and cook, stirring, until softened. Move to a large bowl.

2. Add the lamb, shallots, bread crumbs, parsley, egg, and lemon zest to the bowl. Season with pepper, salt, and marjoram. Store in the refrigerator for one hour.

3. In a skillet set over medium-high heat, melt half of the butter and warm the olive oil. Shape the lamb mixture into little meatballs and sear them in batches in the skillet until they are uniformly browned. Don't empty the skillet. Place the meatballs in a serving dish after draining them on paper towels.

4. Add the wine, cinnamon, garlic, and tomato sauce to the skillet. Cook, stirring, until well heated and well combined. Cover the meatballs with a drizzle of the mixtures.

MY OBSERVATIONS

Asian Beef and Broccoli Stir-Fry

  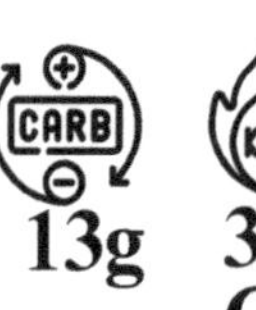 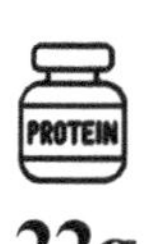 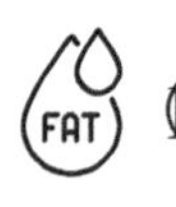 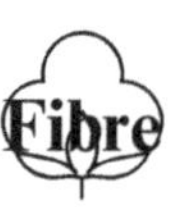 

Prep	Cook	CARB	KCAL	PROTEIN	FAT	Fibre	Servings
15 mins	15 mins	13g	331 Cal	22g	21g	3g	4

Ingredients

- 1 tsp cornstarch
- Cut a ¾-pound beef round steak into strips that are 1/8-inch thick.
- 3 tsp vegetable oil, plus extra if necessary
- 1 small slice of raw ginger
- 1 peeled and smashed garlic clove
- 1 pound of floret-cut broccoli
- One-third cup oyster sauce
- One-third cup sherry
- A couple of tsp of toasted sesame oil
- 1 tsp soy sauce
- 1 tsp white sugar

Instructions

1. In a bowl, combine the oyster sauce, sherry, sesame oil, soy sauce, sugar, and cornstarch; whisk until the sugar is dissolved.

2. Slide the meat into a small bowl. After coating the meat with the oyster sauce mixture and covering it, let it marinade for at least half an hour in the fridge.

3. In a wok or sizable skillet, heat the vegetable oil over medium-high heat. To flavor the oil, add the ginger and garlic, then remove and discard after they have sizzled for about a minute. Add broccoli and stir. For five to seven minutes, toss and mix until brilliant green and almost soft. Take out and place aside the broccoli from the wok.

4. If necessary, add a small amount additional oil to the pan before adding the marinated beef.

5. Stir and toss for approximately five minutes, or until sauce thickens,Add the broccoli back to the wok and stir for three minutes, or until heated throu

MY OBSERVATIONS

Tomato Greek Salad

  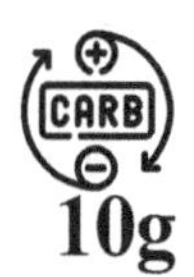 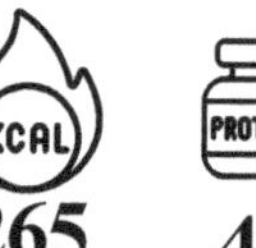 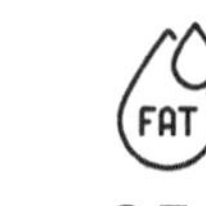 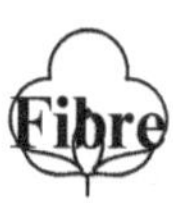 

Prep	Cook	CARB	KCAL	PROTEIN	FAT	Fibre	Servings
15 mins	15 mins	10g	265 Cal	4g	25g	2g	8

Ingredients

- 4 big tomatoes, sliced into wedges
- 1 cucumber, cut in half lengthwise and then sliced
- Chop one-half red onion
- ½ cup black Greek olives
- 1/2 tsp finely chopped fresh basil
- 1/4 tsp finely chopped fresh oregano
- Half a cup of feta cheese, crumbled
- 1 bottle (16 fl oz) of Greek salad dressing
- 1/4 tsp finely ground black pepper
- 1 fresh basil sprig

Instructions

1. In a big bowl, gently combine tomatoes, cucumber, red onion, olives, 1/4 teaspoon minced basil, and oregano; sprinkle feta cheese on top. Drizzle salad with Greek dressing and add a dash of black pepper. Add a fresh basil leaf as a salad garnish.

MY OBSERVATIONS

Pizza Salad

  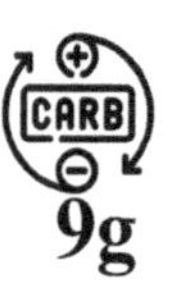  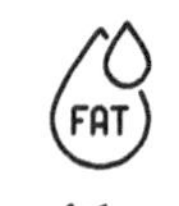 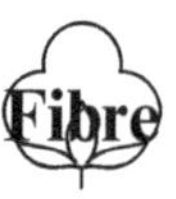 

Prep	Cook	CARB	KCAL	PROTEIN	FAT	Fibre	Servings
15 mins	15 mins	9g	476 Cal	20g	41g	2g	6

Ingredients

- 1 head of iceberg lettuce, shredded into small pieces
- Cut ½ pound of salami into strips.
- 1 cup of finely shredded mozzarella cheese
- 1 cup of cheddar cheese, shredded
- 1 chopped tomato
- halved and pitted ½ cup of black olives
- 1 tablespoon of freshly cut chives
- Dressing Pizza:
- 1 eight-oz can of tomato sauce
- 1/2 cup of vegetable oil & white vinegar
- 1tsp of dehydrated oregano
- 1 tsp salt
- 2 teaspoon of powdered garlic
- 1 tsp finely ground black pepper

Instructions

1. In a big bowl, mix together lettuce, salami, tomato, olives, Cheddar cheese, mozzarella cheese, and chives. Toss to blend well.

2. Apply makeup: In a medium-sized bowl, whisk together tomato sauce, oil, vinegar, sugar, oregano, salt, garlic powder, and pepper.

3. After coating the lettuce mixture with enough dressing, stir and serve.

MY OBSERVATIONS

Salmon Quinoa Bowl

  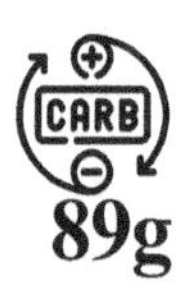  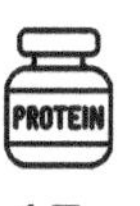 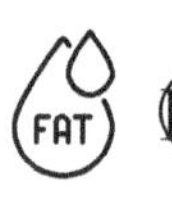 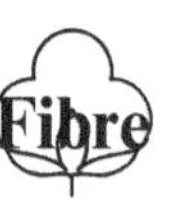 

Prep	Cook	CARB	KCAL	PROTEIN	FAT	Fibre	Servings
15 mins	15 mins	89g	758 Cal	45g	25g	15g	4

Ingredients

- One cup of white quinoa
- 1/4 cup of water
- Half a cup of Greek yogurt
- half a cup tahini
- 1 tablespoon of lemon juice
- 1/4 tsp finely chopped garlic
- 3 tsp water, or more if necessary
- A smidgeon of kosher salt
- 1 ½ packages (8 ounces) lacinato kale
- 2 carrots
- Two fifteen-ounce cans of rinsed and drained chickpeas
- Half a cup of dehydrated cherries
- 1 tablespoon of olive oil
- 4 skin-on (4-ounce) salmon fillets

Instructions

1. In a medium saucepan, combine the quinoa and water; heat to medium-high and bring to a boil. Cook, covered, over medium-low heat for about 12 minutes, or until tender. Take off the heat and leave covered for three to five minutes. Put aside.

2. For the salad, combine yogurt, tahini, lemon juice, and garlic in a big bowl. One tablespoon at a time, add water until the required consistency is achieved. Add some salt for seasoning. Put aside.

3. Remove the kale stalks. Tear the leaves and add them to the dressing-filled basin. Add carrots to the bowl after slicing them into long ribbons. For approximately a minute, massage the dressing into the salad until it is evenly coated. Add the cherries and chickpeas to the kale and mix to coat.

4. In a big, nonstick skillet, heat the oil over medium heat. Sear salmon skin-side down for 4 minutes or until it's

crisp. Turn and continue cooking for another 3 to 4 minutes for medium-rare, or until desired level of doneness is achieved. Transfer to a plate.

5.Split the quinoa among four bowls. Top with salmon and add kale salad. Drizzle some olive oil over the top, sprinkle some black pepper on top, and serve right away.

MY OBSERVATIONS

Adzuki Bean Meatballs

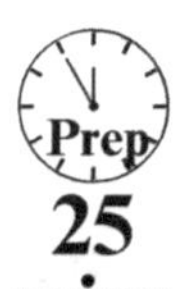 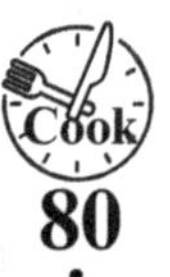 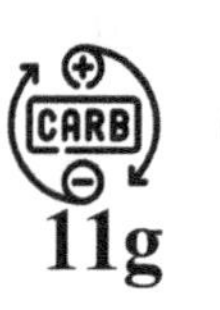 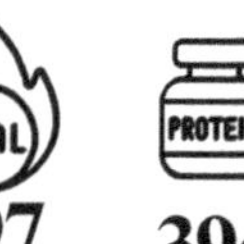 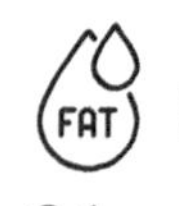 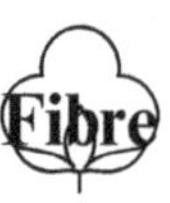 

Prep	Cook	CARB	KCAL	PROTEIN	FAT	Fibre	Servings
25 mins	80 mins	11g	497 Cal	39g	31g	2g	24

Ingredients

- 1 cup of raw adzuki beans, soaked for at least 8 hours, well washed, and then drained; or use 2 cups of cooked adzuki beans.
- 1 medium onion
- 1 medium-sized carrot
- 1/2 cup of basil
- 1/2 cup of pecans
- 1/4 cup organic oats, 1 tsp dry oregano
- One tsp salt
- 1/2 Tsp of pepper, black
- 400 grams/14 oz of crushed tomatoes
- 1 little onion, diced finely
- 3 garlic cloves, cut well
- 1/4 cup chopped coarsely basil plus some for serving
- 1/2 cup of water
- 2 Tsp of olive oil
- 1/2 Tsp of salt
- 1/2 Tsp of pepper, black

Instructions

1. To cook the adzuki beans, put them in a pot with lots of water, just like you would pasta. It's critical to keep in mind that adding salt will cause the bean to cook more slowly and become rigid. Boil for 40 minutes and then continue to cook. Empty.

2. Set aside a large oven tray that has been lined with baking paper or a silicone roasting mat and preheat the oven to 350°F/180°C.

3. All of the meatball ingredients—cooked adzuki beans, onion, carrot, basil, nuts, oats, dried oregano, salt, and pepper—should be combined in a food processor and thoroughly ground until a uniform texture is achieved.

4. Form the meatballs into about 2-inch (5 cm) diameter balls with clean hands. For fifteen minutes, bake them on the baking sheet.

5. Olive oil should be heated in a large sauté pan before adding the finely chopped onion and stirring for two to

three minutes. After a minute, add the chopped garlic cloves and continue cooking. Add the smashed tomatoes, water, salt, pepper, and basil leaves. After bringing to a boil, reduce heat, and simmer for ten minutes. You can add an additional 7 oz (200 grams) of crushed tomatoes and half a cup of water if you want the patties to have a lot of sauce.

6.Gently combine the prepared sauce with the baked patties and heat for an additional five minutes, but not more. Make sure the sauce is simmering rather than boiling before adding the burgers. When serving, scatter some basil leaves on top.

MY OBSERVATIONS

Grilled Chicken Salad

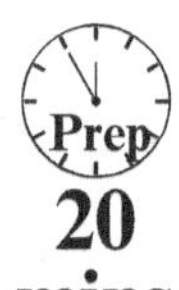  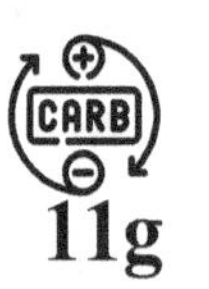 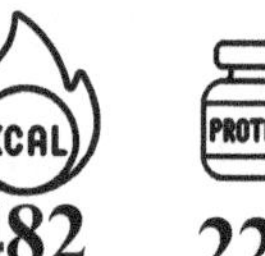 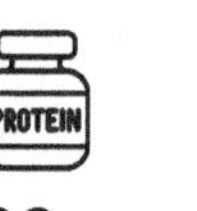 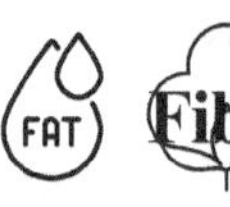 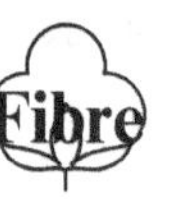 

Prep	Cook	CARB	KCAL	PROTEIN	FAT	Fibre	Servings
20 mins	15 mins	11g	482 Cal	22g	23g	4g	6

Ingredients

- 1-pound chicken breasts, deboned and skinless
- 6 cups of chopped romaine lettuce
- Cherry tomatoes, 3/4 cup
- 3/4 cup fresh (thawed from frozen or canned) corn kernels
- 3/4 cup sliced cucumber
- 1/4 cup sliced red onion
- 1/2 cup fried bacon in crumbles
- 1/2 cup of shredded blue cheese
- Peel, sliced, pit avocado.
- 3 tsp lemon juice
- 2 tsp Dijon mustard
- 3 tsp of vinegar made from red wine
- 2 tsp of powdered sugar
- 2 tsp of shallot, chopped
- 2 tsp dried oregano and parsley
- 1/3 cup olive oil, to taste with salt and pepper

Instructions

1. In a medium-sized bowl, add all the ingredients and whisk until thoroughly mixed.
2. Transfer half of the dressing to a jar so you may use it later.
3. Pour the remaining dressing into the bowl and add the chicken breasts. Let it marinate for one hour or up to eight hours
4. Set a medium-high heat on an indoor or outdoor grill. After removing it from the marinade, put the chicken on the grill.
5. Cook for 5 to 6 minutes on each side, or until chicken is cooked through and browned.
6. After letting the chicken cool for five minutes, slice it.
7. Put the greens into a big basin. Over the lettuce, drizzle half of the saved dressing.
8. On top of the lettuce, arrange the chicken, tomatoes, corn, cucumber, red onion, bacon, blue cheese, and avocado. Pour the remaining dressing over the top and serve right away.

MY OBSERVATIONS

Shrimp and Avocado Sushi Bowls

 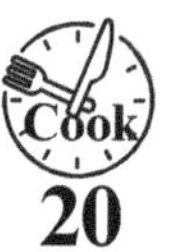 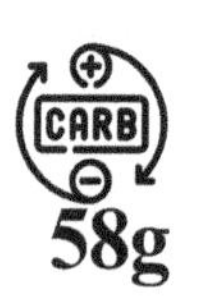 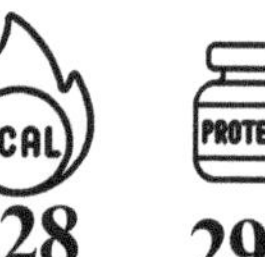 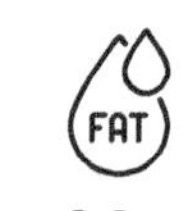 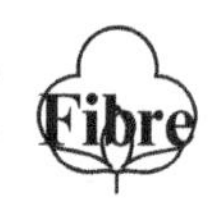 

Prep	Cook	CARB	KCAL	PROTEIN	FAT	Fibre	Servings
15 mins	20 mins	58g	628 Cal	29g	30g	6g	2

Ingredients

- 10 ounces of peeled and deveined tail-on shrimp
- ½ cup of sushi rice
- 2 Persian cucumbers
- 3 ounces of radishes
- 1 Avocado
- 1 tsp of Yuzu Kosho
- 1 tsp of mirin (salted cooking wine)
- 1 tsp of sesame oil
- 1 tsp each of black and white sesame seeds
- 1 tsp of seasoned black vinegar and 2 tablespoons of mayonnaise

Instructions

1. The rice, 3/4 cup water, and a generous teaspoon of salt should all be combined in a small pot. Turn the heat up to boiling. Once boiling, turn down the heat. For 15 to 17 minutes, or until the water has been absorbed and the rice is soft, cover and cook without stirring. Switch off the heat source and use a fork to mix in the mirin.

2. Pit and halve the avocado. After removing the avocado from its peel with a spoon, thinly slice it. Transfer to a bowl and add salt and pepper to taste. Slice the radishes thinly crosswise after halving them lengthwise. Slice the cucumbers thinly crosswise after halving them lengthwise. Sesame oil, vinegar, cucumber slices, and radishes should all be combined in a bowl. Add pepper and salt for seasoning. Allow it to marinade for at least ten minutes, stirring from time to time. To make the dish as spicy as you like, mix the mayonnaise with as much yuzu kosho as you desire in a different bowl.

104

3.Using paper towels, pat the shrimp dry (remove the tails if desired). Add pepper and salt for seasoning. Heat a drizzle of olive oil in a medium pan (nonstick if you have one) over medium-high heat. Stir in the seasoned shrimp. Cook for 4 to 5 minutes, stirring occasionally, or until cooked through and opaque.

4.Switch off the heating source. Serve the cooked rice with the prepared shrimp, seasoned avocado, and marinated veggies (with or without liquid). Pour over the yuzu mayo. Add the sesame seeds as a garnish. Enjoy!

MY OBSERVATIONS

Grilled Veggie and Hummus Wrap

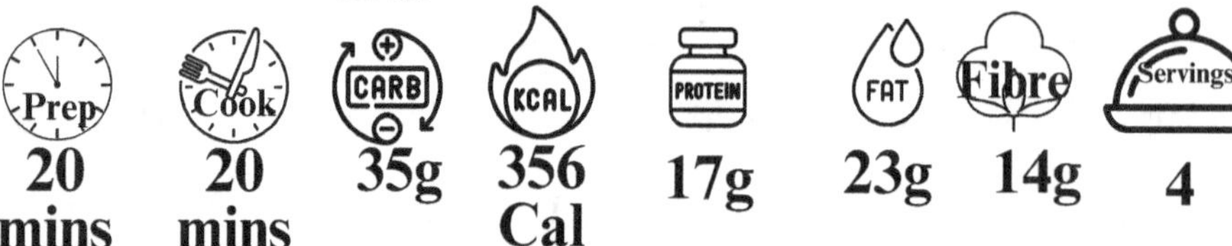

Prep	Cook	CARB	KCAL	PROTEIN	FAT	Fibre	Servings
20 mins	20 mins	35g	356 Cal	17g	23g	14g	4

Ingredients

- Four half-inch-thick red onion slices
- One red bell pepper, cut into quarters and seeds
- One 12-oz eggplant, sliced into half-inch thick pieces
- Two tsp olive oil, separated
- ¼ cup of freshly cut flat-leaf parsley
- 1/4 tsp kosher salt
- One 8-oz container of basic hummus
- Four (1.9-ounce) flatbreads made entirely of grains (like Flatout Light)
- ½ cup of feta cheese in crumbles
- Lettuce with Avocado and Butter

Instructions

1. A large grill pan should be heated at medium-high heat. Apply one tablespoon of oil to the bell pepper, eggplant, and onion. When grill marks start to show, add the onion and bell pepper to the pan and cook for 3 minutes on each side. Take out of the pan. Place eggplant in pan and heat until grill marks form, 3 minutes on each side. Take out of the pan and roughly chop the veggies.

2. Toss to mix the veggies, parsley, salt, and the remaining tablespoon of oil.

3. Leaving a 1/2-inch border around the sides of each flatbread, spread 1/4 cup hummus over them..

4. Top each flatbread with a portion of vegetables and two tablespoons of cheese.

5. Wrap each one, then cut in half on the diagonal.

MY OBSERVATIONS

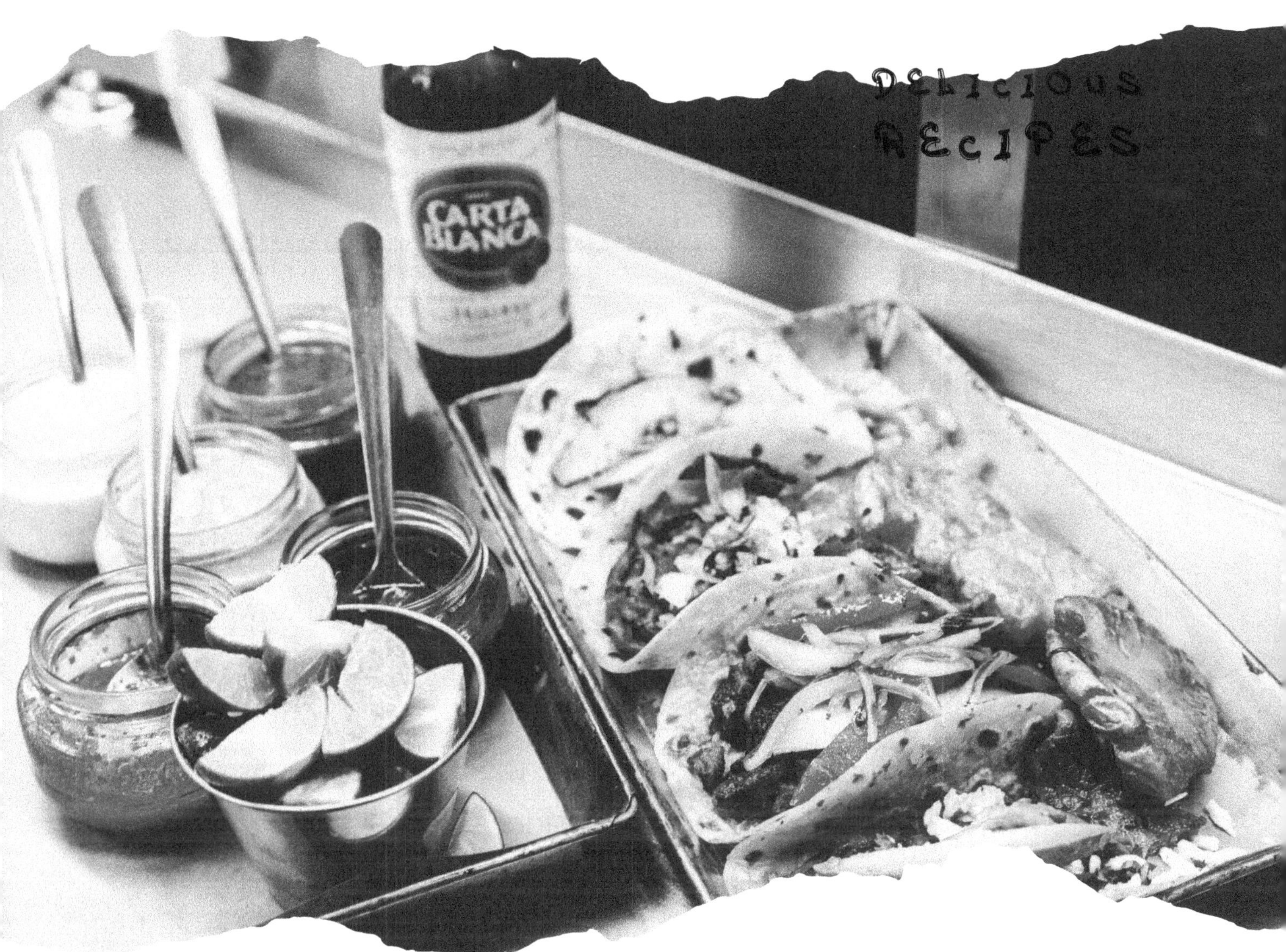

DINNER DINNER DINNER

RECIPES

FOR HEALTHY YOU

Fish Tacos

  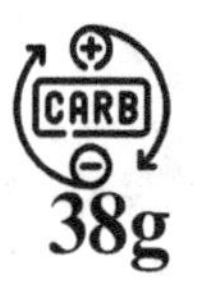  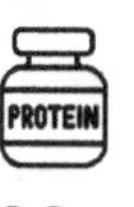 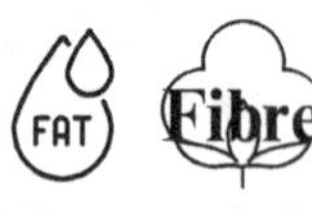 

Prep	Cook	CARB	KCAL	PROTEIN	FAT	Fibre	Servings
15 mins	30 mins	38g	410 Cal	29g	17.4g	6.3g	4

Ingredients

- 1 lime; 1.2 lb/600g firm white fish fillets (Note 1)
- 3 tsp of lime juice
- 1 tsp powdered chipotle
- 1 tsp coarsely chopped canned jalapeño
- 1/4 cup finely chopped cilantro or coriander
- 2 minced cloves of garlic
- 3 tsp of olive oil
- Pepper and salt.
- 4 cups of finely shredded red cabbage
- 3 green onion stalks, cut diagonally and neatly sliced
- 2 tsp of red wine vinegar (or cider vinegar, white wine vinegar)
- 1/2 tsp of salt
- 3/4 cup yogurt or sour cream
- 3 tsp of Sriracha, to taste.

TO PRESENT & COOK

- 1tsp of olive oil
- cilantro/coriander leaves

Instructions

1. Fish marinade: Put all of the ingredients for the marinade in a ziplock bag. Let it marinade for 20 minutes, but no more than an hour.
2. Put the ingredients for the pickled cabbage in a bowl. Mix well and let sit for half an hour. Shake off extra liquid, then use your hands to wriggle the cabbage (to assist soften). Put aside.
3. Blend the pink sauce thoroughly.
4. Cook fish: Place a skillet over high heat with oil. Cook fish until done and golden, 2 minutes per side.
5. Place the fish on a plate and break it up into big chunks.
6. When assembling the tacos, place cabbage, fish, sour cream, and lime juice on top.
7. Enjoy the tortilla after folding it over!

MY OBSERVATIONS

Lemon ginger Salmon

  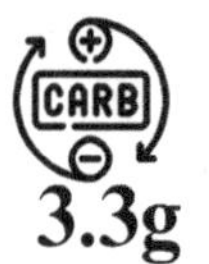  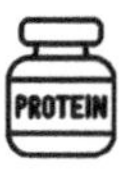 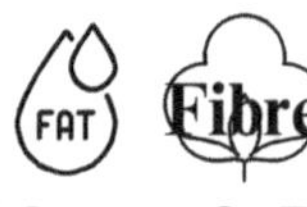 

Prep	Cook	CARB	KCAL	PROTEIN	FAT	Fibre	Servings
15 mins	20 mins	3.3g	391 Cal	64g	12.1g	0.5g	4

Ingredients

- 4 Salmon fillets
- 2 Green onions
- 1 ½ tablespoons finely chopped fresh gingerroot
- 1 minced garlic clove and two tablespoons of low-sodium soy sauce
- 1 tablespoon freshly squeezed lemon juice
- 1 teaspoon each of lemon zest and granulated sugar
- A tablespoon of sesame oil

Instructions

1. Finely chop the green onions. Keep the green tops aside for garnishing.
2. Put the white part of the onions, ginger root, garlic, soy sauce, lemon zest, juice, sugar, and sesame oil in a bowl.
3. In a shallow baking dish, arrange the salmon fillets in a single layer. After applying the marinade, leave it for 15 minutes at room temperature or for 1 hour in the refrigerator.
4. Turn the oven on to 425°F.
5. Bake the salmon for 13 to 15 minutes, uncovered, or until it becomes opaque.
6. Add the saved green onions as a garnish. Furthermore, sesame seeds are a lovely garnish.
7. Instead of baking the salmon in the oven, it might be grilled.

MY OBSERVATIONS

Spring Pesto Pasta

  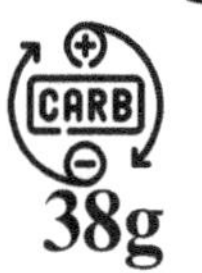  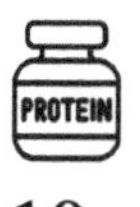 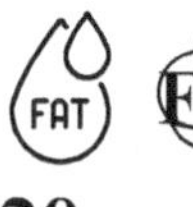 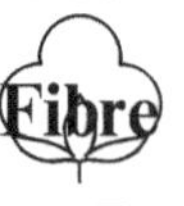 

Prep	Cook	CARB	KCAL	PROTEIN	FAT	Fibre	Servings
15 mins	20 mins	38g	385 Cal	10g	20g	17g	4

Ingredients

- 500g spiralized pasta
- One cup of frozen peas
- 1/2 cup light mayonaise
- 135g piece of Lisa's Pesto Dip with Parmesan, Basil, and Cashews, x1
- One tsp of lemon juice
- 200g of cherry tomatoes
- One spring onion, cut thinly
- one lemon's zest
- fresh basil leaves for decorating

Instructions

1. Pasta should be cooked in a big saucepan as directed on the package until it is al dente. In the final minute of cooking, add the frozen peas to thoroughly heat them through. After draining, set aside to prepare the dressing.

2. Mix the mayonnaise, pesto dip, and lemon juice in a big bowl until well blended. Stir to coat the cooked pasta and peas in the dressing.

3. Mix one more after adding the tomatoes, spring onions, and lemon zest. Transfer into a serving bowl and top with chopped fresh basil.

4. Warm up and serve immediately, or refrigerate until ready to serve.

MY OBSERVATIONS

Shrimp and Veggie Skewers with Quinoa

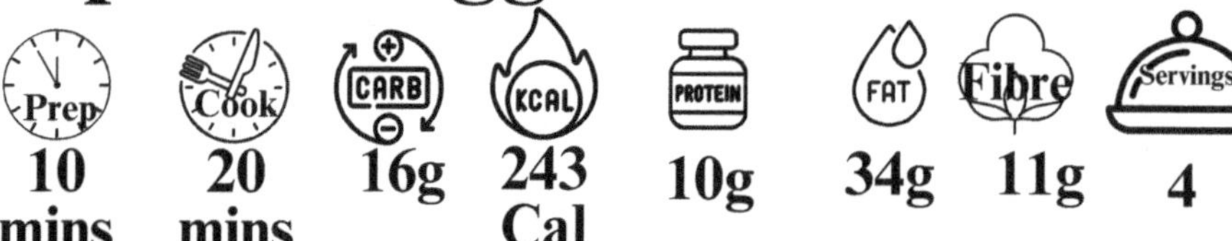

Prep	Cook	CARB	KCAL	PROTEIN	FAT	Fibre	Servings
10 mins	20 mins	16g	243 Cal	10g	34g	11g	4

Ingredients

- 1 tsp of oregano
- 1 pound of raw shrimp
- Blade A: 2 medium zucchini, with trimmed noodles
- 1 cup of cherry tomatoes
- 1 cup of cooked quinoa
- 1/3 cup of feta crumbles
- To serve, quarter one lemon.
- Salt, pepper, and 2 tsp of extra virgin olive oil
- one-half teaspoon paprika
- One-half teaspoon of powdered garlic

Instructions

1. Combine the oregano, garlic powder, paprika, olive oil, and salt & pepper in a medium-sized bowl. Toss thoroughly to coat after adding the shrimp, zucchini, and tomatoes. Using metal skewers, skewer the shrimp and set aside.

2. After dividing the quinoa among bowls or plates, leave it aside.

3. After bringing a grill pan to a medium-high heat, add the zucchini and tomatoes. Allow zucchini to fry for 5 minutes, stirring periodically, or until charred. While keeping the tomatoes in the pan, divide the zucchini among the quinoa-topped plates.

4. When the shrimp are opaque and shaped like a C, add the skewers to the grill pan and cook for two to three minutes on each side.

5. Spoon the quinoa into individual bowls, then garnish with the tomatoes, zucchini, and shrimp, and finish with feta.

116

MY OBSERVATIONS

Lasagna

  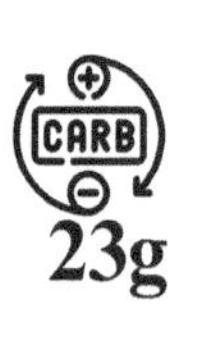  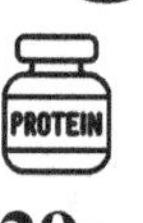 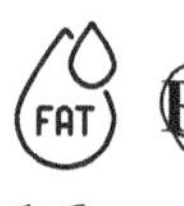 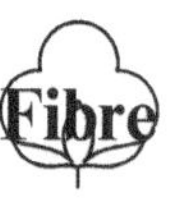 

Prep	Cook	CARB	KCAL	PROTEIN	FAT	Fibre	Servings
30 mins	60 mins	23g	368 Cal	29g	16g	1.1g	12

Ingredients

- 1 pound of ground beef with 15–20% fat
- 1 medium onion, chopped
- 2big cloves of minced garlic
- 1/4 cup beef broth or dry red wine
- One tsp of olive oil
- 3 cups of 24 oz. Marinara sauce
- Half a tsp of sea salt
- 1/4 tsp ground black pepper
- 1/4 tsp of dried thyme
- 1/2 tsp of sugar, granulated
- 2 tsp finely chopped parsley
- 9 lasagna noodles, al dente.

Cheese Sauce Ingredients:

- 16 ounces of low-fat cottage cheese
- 15 ounces of fat-free ricotta cheese , 1 big egg
- 2 tsp coarsely chopped parsley plus more for garnish
- 4 cups of shredded, split mozzarella cheese

Instructions

1. **Meat Sauce**: Add 1 pound of ground beef, diced onion, and 1 tablespoon olive oil to a deep pan or Dutch oven set over medium-high heat. Saute the beef for five minutes, breaking it up, or until the color turns pink. Once aromatic, add the crushed garlic and sauté for an additional minute.

2. Pour in 1/4 cup of wine and stir until almost evaporated, about 2 minutes. Add 3 cups marinara, 2 Tbsp parsley, 1/2 tsp salt, 1/4 tsp pepper, 1/4 tsp thyme, and 1/2 tsp sugar. Once it reaches a simmer, cover and cook for five minutes.

3. **Cheese Sauce:** In a sizable mixing bowl, mix together 16 ounces of cottage cheese, 15 ounces of ricotta, 1 cup of mozzarella, 1 egg, and 2 tablespoons of parsley. Blend thoroughly.

4. For the lasagna, preheat the oven to 375°F. Heat up a big saucepan of water until it boils. Add nine lasagna noodles and salt. As directed on the

packet, cook until firm.

5. Line the bottom of a deep 9x13 casserole dish with 1/2 cup beef sauce. Spread one-third of the meat sauce over three noodles, then top with a cup of mozzarella cheese. Apply and distribute half of your cheese sauce over the dish.

6. Continue until you have three noodle layers: Pour in 1/3 meat sauce, 1 cup mozzarella cheese, 1/2 cheese sauce, and 3 noodles.

7. Add the remaining 1/3 of the meat sauce, 3 noodles, and 1 cup of mozzarella.

8. To prevent the foil from clinging to the cheese, pierce the top of the lasagna with nine to twelve toothpicks. Bake for 45 minutes at 375°F with the foil covering.

9. Take off the foil and broil the cheese for 3 to 5 minutes, until it becomes brown. Give lasagna 30 minutes to rest before cutting.

MY OBSERVATIONS

Moroccan Lamb Tagine

  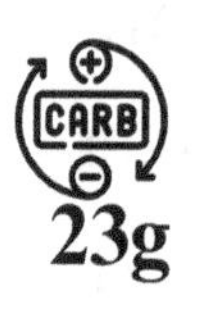  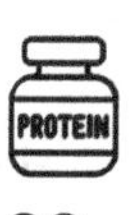 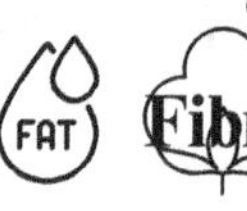 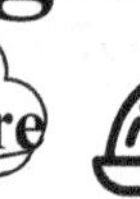 

Prep	Cook	CARB	KCAL	PROTEIN	FAT	Fibre	Servings
30 mins	60 mins	23g	368 Cal	29g	16g	1.1g	12

Ingredients

- Slice a 4-pound boneless lamb roast into 1-inch slices.
- Three c. low-sodium chicken broth and Kosher salt
- 1. Dried apricots
- Three tsp extra virgin olive oil
- one medium onion diced and four sliced garlic cloves
- 2 tsp finely chopped, ginger
- TWO TBC of tomato paste
- 1 cinnamon stick
- A little saffron pinch
- 1½ tsp of ground turmeric
- Grind 1/2 tsp of coriander, cardamom, 1/4 tsp
- 1/4 tsp. nutmeg powder
- 1/4 teaspoon powdered cloves
- freshly ground black pepper
- 1/4 cup of finely chopped cilantro, with additional for decoration
- Half a cup of roasted almond shards
- Tear of mint leaves, to serve.
- Prepared couscous to served

Instructions

1. Toss lamb with approximately 2 teaspoons of salt in a big bowl. Store in the refrigerator overnight or for one hour at room temperature.

2. Heat the chicken broth in a small saucepan over medium-high heat. Take off the heat and stir in the dried apricots. Give it a minimum of fifteen minutes.

3. Heat the oil in a tagine or Dutch oven over medium-high heat. Add the lamb and cook for 4 minutes on each side, or until golden. As needed, work in batches. Take out the lamb and set it onto a platter.

4. Add the onion to the pot and lower the heat to medium. Cook for 5 minutes, or until tender. Add the ginger and garlic and cook for an additional minute or until fragrant, then add the tomato paste and stir until well coated.Cook for an additional minute after adding the spices, saffron, and cinnamon stick until toasted.

5. Fill the pot with the lamb, apricots, and broth; season with salt and pepper. Bring to a boil, then lower the heat and simmer, covered, for about 1½ hours, or until the lamb is tender and the liquid has reduced.

.6. Take off from heat and add the cilantro. Add some more cilantro, mint, and toasted almonds as garnish. Toss with warm couscous.

MY OBSERVATIONS

Turkey and Vegetable Stir-Fry with Brown Rice

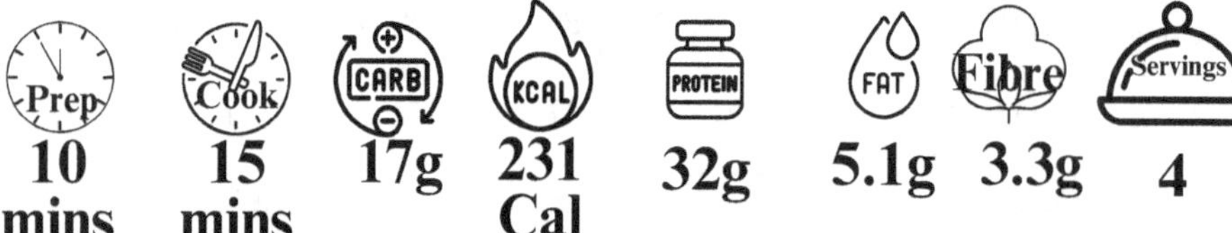

Ingredients

- 1 medium onion, chopped
- 1 pound of ground turkey breast
- 2 grated garlic cloves
- 1 tsp grated ginger
- One-half tsp each of salt and pepper
- 1 cup of low-sodium chicken broth
- 2 tsp of low-sodium soy sauce
- 1 tsp of vinegar made from rice wine
- 1 tsp of paste with chilies
- 1 tsp of corn flour
- 1 tsp of hoisin sauce
- 4 cups florets of broccoli
- ½ cup finely chopped scallions

Instructions

1. Apply nonstick spray to a sizable, deep pan and place it on medium-high heat.

2. Add the onions and cook for 3–4 minutes, or until soft.

3. In the meantime, combine the broth, soy sauce, rice wine vinegar, corn starch, chili garlic paste, and hoisin sauce in a small bowl. Put aside.

4. To the pan with the onions, add the ground turkey breast, garlic, ginger, salt, and pepper. Cook for 5 to 7 minutes, or until the turkey is browned. The turkey breast can be broken up with a wooden spoon.

5. Add the chicken broth mixture and broccoli florets once the turkey has browned. Bring to a boil and cover and simmer until broccoli is tender, about 6 minutes. Add some scallions to the brown rice that has been cooked with green peas, sesame oil, and scallions right before serving.

MY OBSERVATIONS

Pasta Carbonara with Crispy Kale

  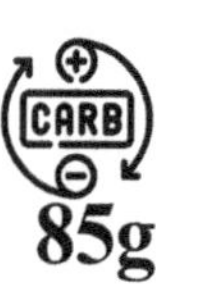 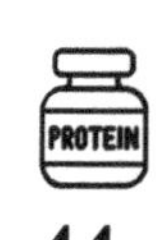 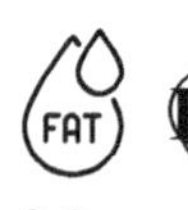 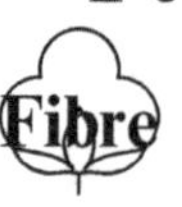 

Prep	Cook	CARB	KCAL	PROTEIN	FAT	Fibre	Servings
15 mins	15 mins	85g	899 Cal	44g	39g	14g	2

Ingredients

- 200g curly kale, roughly torn, with hard stalks removed; 3 tablespoons olive oil, plus an additional splash
- hefty pinch of salt flakes
- 200g of spiral pasta, such as bucatini
- 3 medium-sized, organic eggs
- 70g of grated Parmesan cheese or a vegetarian substitute, plus additional to serve
- 1 onion, chopped finely
- 3 large cloves of finely chopped garlic

Instructions

1. Set oven temperature to 180°C fan/gas 6. Toss the kale thoroughly after adding 2 tablespoons of oil and salt to a large bowl. Arrange the kale evenly among one or two baking trays and bake for five minutes, or until crisp (watch it closely to avoid burning). Put aside to cool.

2. Cook the pasta until it's al dente, or just slightly bite-sized, following the directions on the package. After draining, set aside 100ml of pasta water, and toss the pasta in a little oil to prevent it from sticking together.

3. In a small bowl, beat together the eggs, parmesan, a dash of salt, and a generous amount of black pepper to create the carbonara sauce. Finally, add a splash of the pasta water that was set aside. Put aside.

4. In a large, nonstick frying pan, warm up the remaining oil and sauté the onion for four to five minutes over medium heat. Cook for one more minute after adding the garlic and

most of the pasta water that was set aside.

5. Reduce the heat to low and add the carbonara sauce mixture after tossing the cooked pasta with the peas in the pan. After a minute of vigorous stirring over low heat, add a little more pasta water to loosen. Serve with extra Parmesan and black pepper after tossing in the crispy kale.

MY OBSERVATIONS

Spicy Seafood

  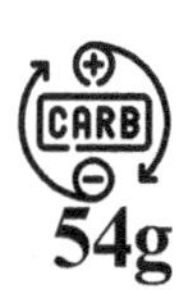  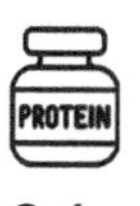 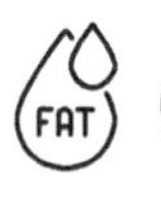 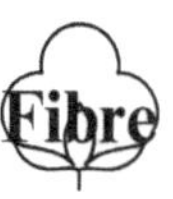 

Prep	Cook	CARB	KCAL	PROTEIN	FAT	Fibre	Servings
15 mins	20 mins	54g	444 Cal	34g	10g	3.8g	4

Ingredients

- 8 ounces of raw linguine
- 2 tsp extra virgin olive oil, split
- Half a pound of bay scallops
- 6 ounces of medium shrimp, peeled and deveined
- ½ cup finely chopped onion
- 1/4 to 1/2 tsp finely ground red pepper
- 3 minced garlic cloves
- 2 tsp of tomato paste
- 1 14.5-oz can of diced tomatoes, drained and petite-cut
- half a cup of clam juice
- 12 littleneck clams
- 12 mussels, cleaned and without beards
- 2 tablespoons of freshly chopped parsley
- 1 tablespoon of fresh basil, thinly sliced

Instructions

1. Cook pasta as directed on the package, leaving out the fat and salt; drain.

2. While the pasta cooks, place a large nonstick skillet over medium-high heat with 1 tablespoon of oil. Cook the shrimp and scallops in the pan for three minutes. Take out of the pan the scallop mixture and keep it warm. In the pan, heat the remaining tablespoon of oil over medium-high heat. Add the garlic, onion, and red pepper; cook for two minutes. After adding the tomatoes and tomato paste, boil for two minutes. Stir in clam juice and cook for 1 minute. Cover, lower the heat to medium, and cook the clams for 4 minutes. When the clams and mussels open, add the mussels, cover, and cook for three minutes. Throw away any unopened casings. Add the parsley and scallop mixture, and cook for 1 minute, or until heated through. Turn over pasta, Sprinkle Basil.

126

MY OBSERVATIONS

Baked Salmon with Quinoa and Steamed Asparagus

  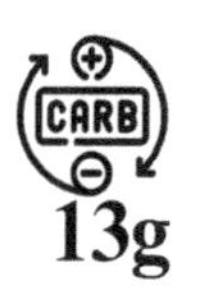 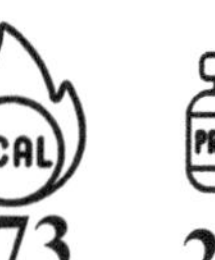 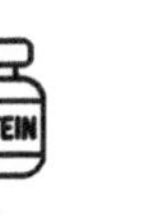 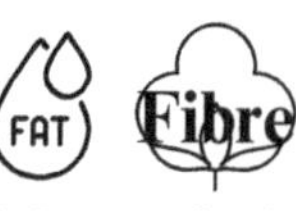 

Prep	Cook	CARB	KCAL	PROTEIN	FAT	Fibre	Servings
20 mins	25 mins	13g	573 Cal	29g	12g	3.1g	2

Ingredients

- 5 tsp of lemon juice
- 1 tsp of Dijon mustard
- 1 tsp of agave
- 1 of olive oil
- 1 tiny shallot, chopped finely
- 1 tsp of freshly chopped dill
- Add pepper and salt.
- 1 tsp of olive oil
- 1 chopped shallot
- half a cup of quinoa
- 1 cup of chicken broth
- If necessary, add salt and pepper.
- Avocado and Salmon
- 2 8-oz skinless salmon fillets that are ½ inch thick
- 1 tsp of olive oil
- 3 sliced garlic cloves
- 1 tsp of butter without salt
- 8 ounces of trimmed, thick asparagus
- Add pepper and salt.

Instructions

1. First, make the dressing. In a small bowl, whisk together agave, lemon juice, Dijon mustard, and olive oil. Add the dill and shallot. To taste, add salt and pepper for seasoning. Put aside.

2. Cook the pilaf of quinoa. Add the oil and shallot to a small pot. Simmer for two minutes, or until tender. For a further two minutes, add the quinoa and sauté. Simmer after adding the broth. Once the quinoa has formed craters and most of the liquid has been absorbed, cover, lower the heat to low, and cook for 14 to 15 minutes. Switch off the heating source. Replace the lid after covering with a fresh, thin kitchen towel. This will maintain its warmth and fluff while you cook the remaining ingredients.

3. As the quinoa cooks, use paper towels to pat the salmon dry and season it lightly on both sides with salt and pepper. In a nonstick skillet, heat oil over medium-high heat until it begins

128

to smoke slightly. Depending on the size and thickness of your fillets, cook them in a skillet for three to five minutes, or until they are browned on the first side. Flip fillets gently. Lower the heat to medium and cook for another two to four minutes, or until the fish is flaky but still pink and translucent in the center when tested for medium-rare. When ready to serve, transfer to a plate and cover loosely with aluminum foil to keep warm.

4. Garlic slices should be added to the remaining oil in the pan and cooked over medium heat until fragrant and golden brown. Slice the garlic and place it on a plate covered with paper towels. With the tips pointing in one direction, add half of the asparagus spears to the skillet and the remaining spears with the tips pointing in the other direction.

5. After adding salt, cover. Cook for 2 to 3 minutes, depending on the thickness of the asparagus, or until the spears are crisp but have browned on one side. After a minute, or until the food is crisp-tender, uncover and continue to stir. Place a heaping serving of quinoa pilaf on each plate. Top with the salmon fillets. Arrange the asparagus pieces on the side and drizzle with the herb dressing. Arrange reserved on top of asparagus

MY OBSERVATIONS

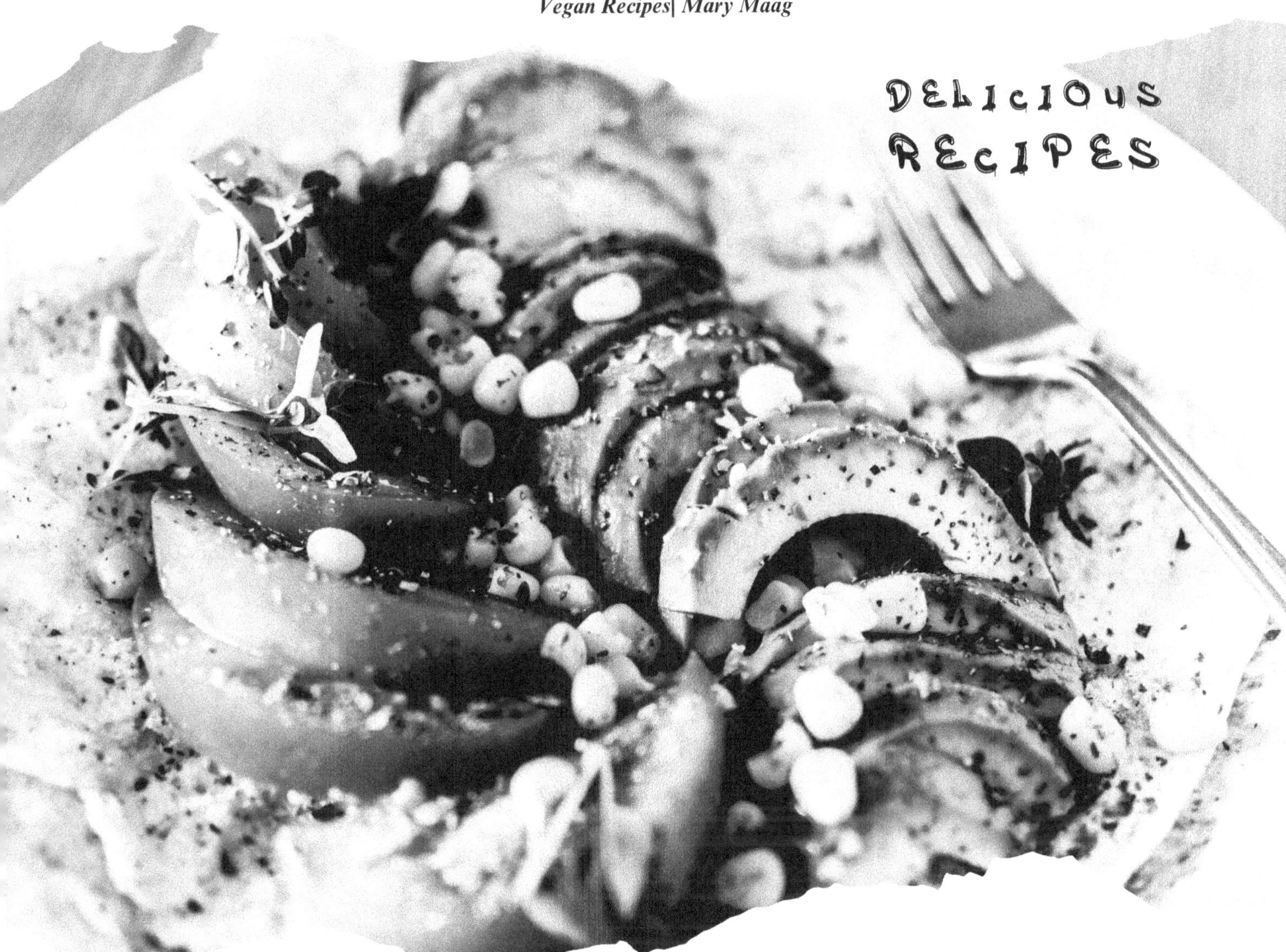

VEGAN

VEGAN **VEGAN** VEGAN

RECIPES

FOR HEALTHY YOU

131

Vegan Lentil Shepherd's Pie

  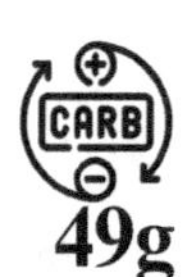  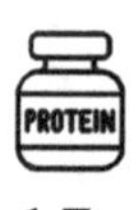 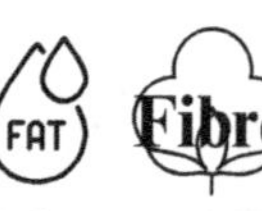 

Prep	Cook	CARB	KCAL	PROTEIN	FAT	Fibre	Servings
17 mins	90 mins	49g	366 Cal	15g	12g	15g	8

Ingredients

Filling with Lentils

- 1 tsp of olive oil
- 8 minced garlic cloves (use less if you're not a big fan of garlic) and three large yellow onions, chopped
- 1 tsp of freshly chopped, coarsely chopped thyme
- 2 tsp finely chopped fresh rosemary leaves
- Tomato paste, 3 tsp
- A half-cup (120 mL) of dry red wine, like Malbec or Pinot Noir One and a half cups (10 ounces / 285g) brown or green lentils
- 900 milliliters, or 3 3/4 cups vegetable stock
- 2 bay leaves
- 2 tsp hot or sweet paprika
- 1/4 cup (56g) silky tahini
- 1 tsp soy sauce or tamari
- 1 tsp of high-grade balsamic vinegar

Instructions

1. Get the Lentil Filling Ready. In an ovenproof 12-inch skillet set over medium to medium-high heat, warm the olive oil until it's hot. The cooked lentil filling must be transferred to a baking dish for baking if you do not have an ovenproof skillet.

2. After adding the onions and a few pinches of salt, sauté them for eight to ten minutes, or until the majority of the onions have browned. Stir occasionally to keep from burning, but not too frequently to allow for browning. Cook the garlic, thyme, and rosemary for two minutes, stirring often to avoid burning.

3. Leave a space unoccupied in the center of the pan by pushing the onions to its edges. Stir the tomato paste into the empty space for two to three minutes, or until the paste takes on a darker hue. As needed, turn down the heat to medium.

4. Add the red wine and deglaze the pan, scraping up any browned bits as you

132

- 2 tsp vegan Worcestershire sauce (may be substituted)
- Sea salt or kosher salt
- Freshly ground pepper

Mashed Potato Garnishing

- 20 ounces (680 g) russet potatoes
- 16 ounces (454 g) chopped cauliflower into big floretss
- 2 tsp kosher saltl to taste
- 1 sprig of rosemary, optional
- 4 tsp of room-temperature-softened vegan butter (or olive oil)
- 120 mL or half a cup of "lite" coconut milk
- 1 tsp of nutritional yeast

Garnishes(optional)

- Extra virgin olive oil for finishing and baking
- Sea salt and black pepper flake
- Newly harvested thyme leaves
- Parsley, chopped flat leaves

go, for three to four minutes, or until the liquid has mostly evaporated and the alcohol smell has subsided.

5. Stir in the lentils, paprika, bay leaves, and vegetable broth. After combining everything, turn up the heat so it boils.

6. After coming to a boil, lower the heat to maintain a quick simmer and cook for 25 to 30 minutes, or until the lentils are just starting to become soft and most of the liquid has been absorbed.

7. Reduce the temperature. Stir in the vegan Worcestershire sauce, tamari, tahini, and balsamic vinegar (if using).

8. Mix thoroughly until combined. After giving it a taste test, I liberally added black pepper and salt (I used about 1 teaspoon of kosher salt). Put aside.

9. Mash the potatoes to make the topping. After peeling, give the russet potatoes a quick rinse in cold water. Cut potatoes into eighth-size pieces.

10. In a large saucepan or Dutch oven, combine the potatoes and cauliflower florets; add just enough water to cover. Incorporate 1/2 tsp of kosher salt and mix thoroughly. Top with the rosemary sprig. Bring to a boil and cook for 15 minutes or until potatoes and cauliflower are fork-tender and extremely soft.

133

In a colander, thoroughly drain the potatoes and cauliflower and throw away the rosemary sprig. Using paper towels or a fresh dish towel, pat dry the potatoes. Squeeze out excess water from the cauliflower or it will be very watery.

11. You can either move the veggies to a big bowl or back to the saucepan. Add the nutritional yeast, lite coconut milk, softened vegan butter, and salt and black pepper to taste. I use an immersion blender, but you can use a handheld potato masher to mash everything together. If necessary, add more salt after tasting for seasonings (I used about 1 teaspoon of kosher salt).

12. Put the Shepherd's Pie together. Turn the oven on to 375°F, or 190°C. Leave the Lentil Filling in your skillet if it's ovenproof and has enough room. If not, move it to a sizable baking dish (3 quarts/3 liters). Even out the lentil filling. Next, use a spoon to evenly distribute the Mashed Potato Topping across the entire surface. Drizzle extra virgin olive oil and additional pinches of pepper, salt, and fresh thyme leaves over the top for extra flavor.

13. Bake the lentil filling for 20 minutes, or until it begins to bubble. Take out of the oven and activate the broiler on your oven. For a few minutes, or until the crust is golden brown, place the pan under the broiler. Finally, add a final drizzle of olive oil and, if preferred, garnish with fresh parsley.

Note: Let the pie sit in the pan for at least 20 minutes if you would like it to solidify even more.

14. Any leftovers can be kept in the refrigerator for up to four days in an airtight container.

MY OBSERVATIONS

Vegan Lentil Sloppy Joes

  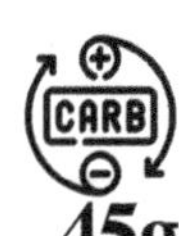  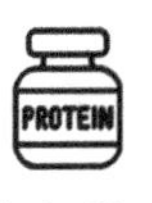 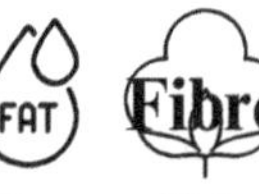 

Prep	Cook	CARB	KCAL	PROTEIN	FAT	Fibre	Servings
5 mins	25 mins	45g	298 Cal	14.8g	8g	17.1g	1

Ingredients

LENTILS

- 2 cups of water
- 1 cup of thoroughly rinsed red or green lentils

SLOPPY JOES

- 2 tsp of avocado, grapeseed, or olive oil
- Minced half a medium white or yellow onion
- 2 minced garlic cloves
- Diced half of a medium red or green bell pepper
- Black pepper and sea salt
- 1 15-ounce can of tomato sauce; 1-2 tsp of coconut sugar
- 1-2 Tbsp vegan Worcestershire sauce (make sure it's gluten-free for people with gluten sensitivity)
- A tsp or two of chili powder
- 1 tsp ground cumin; add more according to taste
- 1 pinch of smoked or regular paprika

Instructions

1. If using green lentils: Rinse the lentils and add the liquid (I used 1 cup water and 1 cup vegetable broth for flavor; use the amount specified in the original recipe; adjust if batch size changes) to a small saucepan. Heat the mixture over medium-high heat. After bringing to a gentle boil, lower the heat to a simmer and cook, covered, for 18 to 22 minutes, or until the food is tender. The water should never boil; it should always simmer. After removing any leftover liquid, set aside.

2. If using red lentils, place liquid (vegetable broth or water) in a small saucepan and heat until it boils. After bringing to a gentle boil, add the rinsed red lentils and continue boiling.

3. Lower the temperature to a simmer and cook, covered, stirring from time to time, for 7 to 10 minutes, until the food is just tender. They should be fully cooked but not mushy. After thorough draining, set aside.

4. Meanwhile, place a big skillet on medium heat. Add the bell pepper, onion, garlic, and oil once heated. Add a small amount of salt and pepper to taste and mix well.

5. Add the peppers and onions and sauté, stirring frequently, for 4–5 minutes, or until soft and lightly browned.

6. Add the vegan Worcestershire sauce, tomato sauce, coconut sugar, cumin, chili powder, and optional paprika next. Mix everything together.

7. Add the cooked lentils to the skillet as well and mix everything together.

8. Stirring occasionally, cook the mixture over medium-low heat for another five to ten minutes, or until it is thickened and thoroughly warmed through.

9. If necessary, add more cumin or chili powder for smokiness, salt for saltiness, coconut sugar for sweetness, or Worcestershire for depth of flavor. Taste and adjust flavor as necessary.

10. Serve the mixture with sliced onion on top of toasted buns. Sloppy Joe mixture is best when fresh, but it can be frozen for a month or kept in the refrigerator for up to 4–5 days. If the mixture has dried out, reheat in the microwave or on the stovetop while adding water or vegetable broth.

MY OBSERVATIONS

Vegan Chickpea Curry

  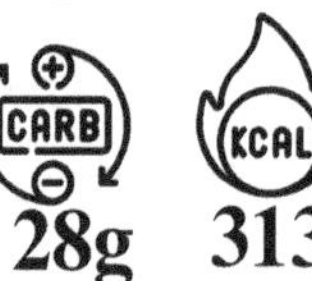 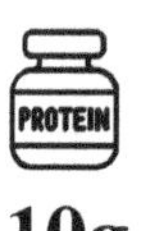 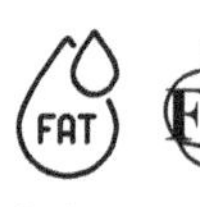 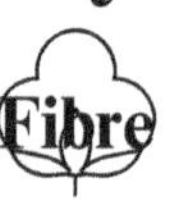 

Prep	Cook	CARB	KCAL	PROTEIN	FAT	Fibre	Servings
10 mins	25 mins	28g	313 Cal	10g	21g	8g	6

Ingredients

- 1 tsp of olive oil
- 1 chopped yellow onion
- 1 minced garlic cloves
- 4 young thyme sprigs
- 1 inch of freshly grated or minced ginger
- Roughly chop 3 medium globe tomatoes.
- 1 tsp each of water and tomato paste
- 2 tsp of curry powder
- 1 tsp of salt
- One-half tsp of all spices
- One-half tsp of ground ginger
- ½ tsp of cumin powder
- 1/2 of garam masala
- One-half tsp of turmeric
- One-third of a tsp red pepper flakes, or to taste
- 15 oz (400 ml) full-fat can of coconut milk
- ½ cup of vegetable stock
- 29 ounces of rinsed and drained chickpeas (878g)
- 3 cup freshly chopped spinach

Instructions

1. Add the oil to a large, high-walled skillet and place it over medium heat. Cook the onion until it becomes tender. Add the ginger, thyme, and garlic and cook for one more minute.

2. Stir in your chopped tomatoes and let them soften for a few minutes. .

3. Mix the tomato paste and water in a small bowl. Combine it with all the spices (red pepper flakes to curry powder) in the skillet and stir to mix. If necessary, add a little oil to help the mixture turn into a paste.

4. Add coconut milk and stock, stirring to fully incorporate the mixture. When the chickpeas are added, simmer. Give the curry a 25-minute simmer to thicken and become creamy.

5. Cook the spinach for 2 minutes, stirring occasionally, until it wilts.

6. Garnish with extra red flakes, chopped red or green onions, and serve alongside rice,naan, quinoa,etc

MY OBSERVATIONS

Quinoa and Black Bean Chili

  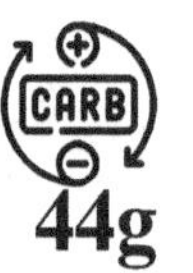  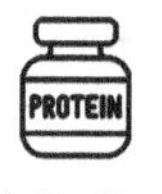 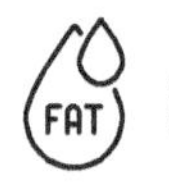 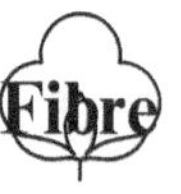 

Prep	Cook	CARB	KCAL	PROTEIN	FAT	Fibre	Servings
17 mins	34 mins	44g	343 Cal	15.3g	8.7g	12.6g	4

Ingredients

- 1 chopped onion
- 2 cloves of garlic, minced
- 1 chopped red pepper
- olive oil spray
- 2 teaspoons of cumin powder
- 1 teaspoon hot smoked paprika
- 1/2 teaspoon red pepper powder (optional)
- 200 g quinoa, rinsed and drained
- 600 ml of vegetable broth
- 400 g crushed tomatoes
- 400 g black beans, washed and drained
- Coriander leaves, to serve

Instructions

1. In olive oil, sauté the onion, garlic, and red pepper until they are soft. If you like your food spicy, add additional spices. After adding the black beans, quinoa, soup, and tomatoes, season to taste. The quinoa should be soft and the sauce should thicken after 30 minutes of simmering under cover.Garnish with some coriander leaves and serve.

MY OBSERVATIONS

Healthy Lentil Tacos

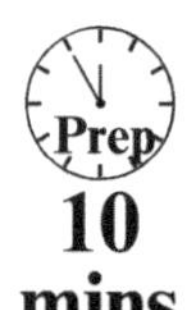  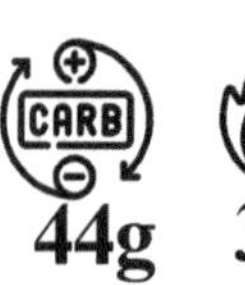 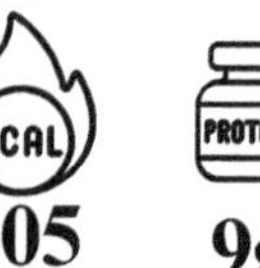 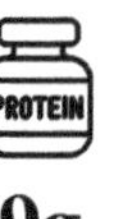 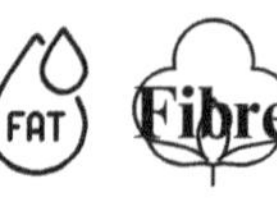 

Prep	Cook	CARB	KCAL	PROTEIN	FAT	Fibre	Servings
10 mins	45 mins	44g	305 Cal	9g	11g	12.9g	6

Ingredients

- 1 teaspoon canola oil
- ⅔ cup finely chopped onion
- 1 small clove of garlic, chopped
- ⅔ cup dry lentils, rinsed
- 1 tablespoon taco seasoning or to taste
- 1 ⅔ cup chicken broth
- ⅔ cup salsa
- 12 taco shells

Instructions

1. Over a medium heat, warm the oil in a skillet. Cook for approximately five minutes, or until the onion and garlic are soft. Stir in lentils and taco seasoning after adding to onion mixture. Stir and cook for 3 minutes or less.

2. Once the chicken broth has been added to the pan, bring it to a boil.

3. Reduce the heat to low, cover the pan, and simmer the lentils for 25 to 30 minutes, or until they are tender. Remove from pan and continue cooking for another 6 to 8 minutes, or until mixture begins to slightly thicken. Grind the lentils to a slightly coarse texture. Pour in the salsa and give it a mix.

4. Place roughly 1/4 cup of the lentil mixture into each taco shell

MY OBSERVATIONS

Buddha Bowls With Shredded Sprouts

  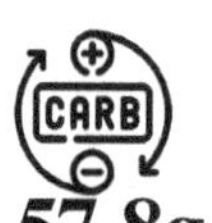  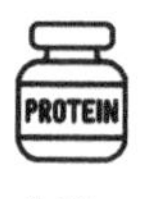 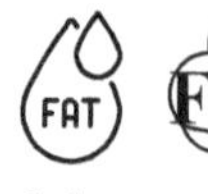 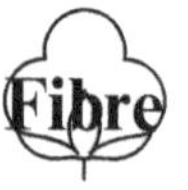 

Prep	Cook	CARB	KCAL	PROTEIN	FAT	Fibre	Servings
10 mins	15 mins	57.8g	428 Cal	18g	11g	14g	4

Ingredients

- olive oil
- 1 lemon, zested and squeezed
- 1 tablespoon Dijon or whole grain mustard
- 400 g cooked quinoa or couscous
- A handful of chopped cilantro and mint
- 2 carrots, peeled and finely chopped
- 400 g chicken breast, rinsed and drained
- 12 Brussels sprouts, trimmed and chopped
- 2 large beets, diced
- 2 red peppers, seeded and finely chopped
- 2 tablespoons toasted sunflower seeds or pumpkin seeds

Instructions

1. Combine one tablespoon of oil, zest, juice, mustard, and seasoning in a whisk. Add the chopped herbs and cooked quinoa to half of the dressing. Divide among four bowls.

2. Top the quinoa with the carrots, beans, bean sprouts, beetroot, and pepper. After adding the remaining vinaigrette and tossing in the seeds, serve.

MY OBSERVATIONS

Miso Soup with Crispy Smoked Tofu

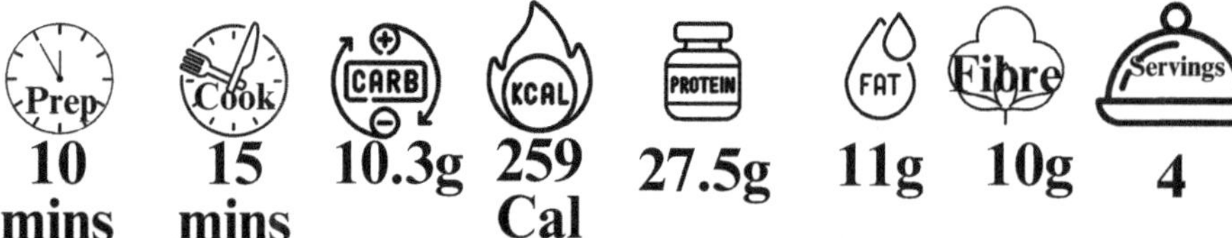

Prep	Cook	CARB	KCAL	PROTEIN	FAT	Fibre	Servings
10 mins	15 mins	10.3g	259 Cal	27.5g	11g	10g	4

Ingredients

- 1 liter of vegetable broth
- 10 g dried shiitake mushrooms
- 2 tablespoons of white soy paste
- Ginger-sized ginger, finely chopped
- 1 clove of garlic, minced
- 100 g smoked tofu, drained and diced
- 2 teaspoons of sesame oil
- 100 grams of garlic
- 2 teaspoons of sesame seeds
- 4 finely chopped seaweed snacks

Instructions

1. Heat the pan slowly after adding the stock, soy paste, ginger, and garlic. Simmer for five minutes.

2. In a skillet, preheat to medium. When the tofu is crispy, add the sesame oil, season, and fry it for four to five minutes.

3. Toss in the kale and cook for 2 to 3 minutes, or until it wilts, in the boiling broth.

4. Transfer the garlic into a large bowl, then top with seaweed, crispy smoked tofu, and sesame seeds.

MY OBSERVATIONS

This page was intentionally left blank.

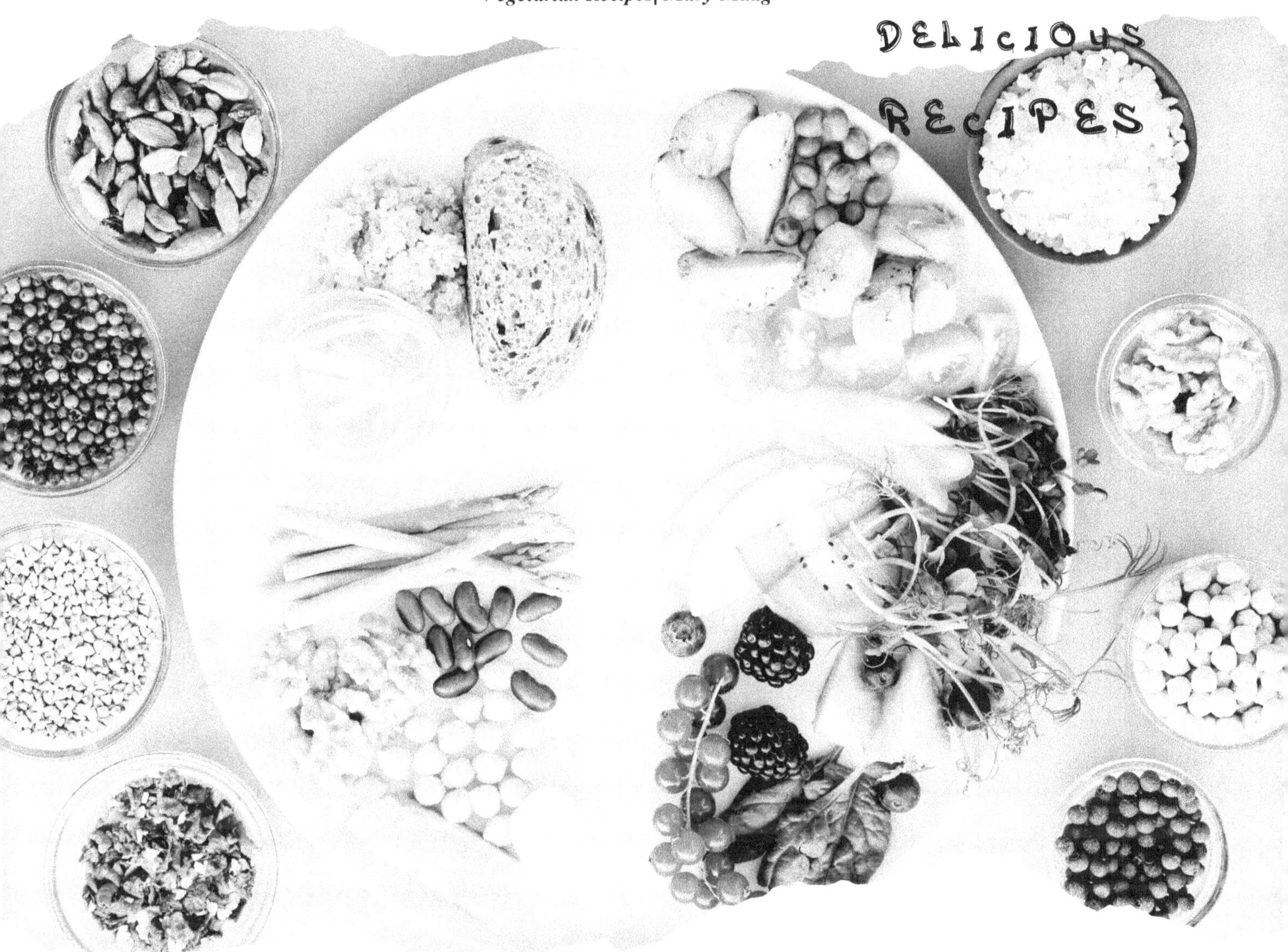

VEGETARIAN
RECIPES

FOR HEALTHY YOU

Butternut Squash Soup

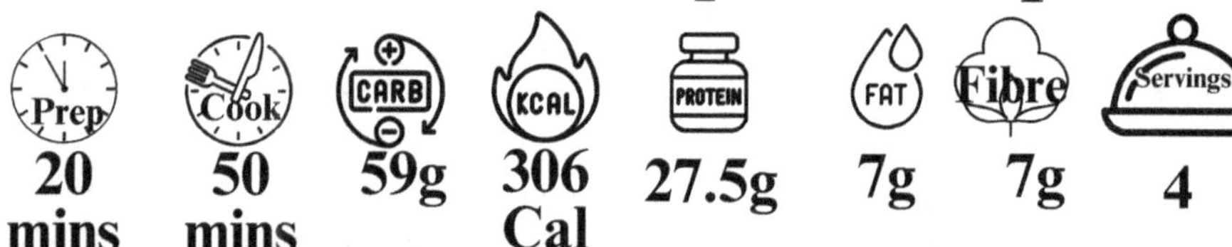

Prep	Cook	CARB	KCAL	PROTEIN	FAT	Fibre	Servings
20 mins	50 mins	59g	306 Cal	27.5g	7g	7g	4

Ingredients

- 2 tablespoons of butter
- 1 small onion, chopped
- 1 stalk of celery, chopped
- 2 medium carrots, finely chopped
- 1 medium butternut squash, peeled, seeded and diced
- 1 container (32 fluid ounces) chicken
- Season with salt and freshly ground pepper.

Instructions

1. Unite the ingredients.
2. Melt the butter in a large saucepan over medium heat, then cook the potatoes, squash, carrots, onions, and celery for about five minutes, or until they are lightly browned.
3. Add enough chicken so that the vegetables are covered. Heat to a boil on a medium-high heat setting. After covering the pot and lowering the heat to low, simmer the vegetables for about 40 minutes, or until they are all tender.
4. Blend the soup in a blender until its smooth. To get the right consistency, return to the saucepan and stir in the remaining ingredients. add salt and pepper for seasoning. Enjoy!

MY OBSERVATIONS

French Onion soup

  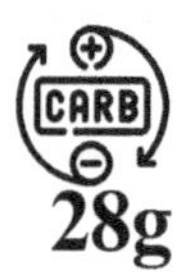  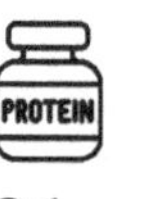 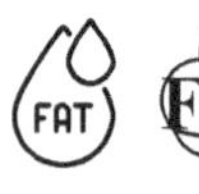 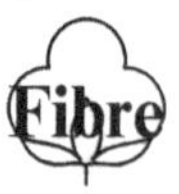 

Prep	Cook	CARB	KCAL	PROTEIN	FAT	Fibre	Servings
15 mins	47 mins	28g	588 Cal	21g	44g	3g	4

Ingredients

- ½ cup unsalted butter
- 2 tablespoons of olive oil
- 4 cups chopped onions
- 5 cups of beef broth
- 2 tablespoons dry sherry
- 1 teaspoon dried thyme
- 1 pinch of salt and pepper to taste
- 4 slices of French bread
- 4 pieces of provolone cheese
- 2 slices of diced Swiss cheese
- ¼ cup grated parmesan

Instructions

1. In an eight-quart pot set over medium heat, melt butter and olive oil.
2. When the onion is soft and transparent, add it to the butter and continue to cook. Avoid letting the onion turn brown.
3. Stir in the sherry, thyme, and beef stock. To season, add your pepper and salt.
4. Place the soup into a baking dish and top with bread, breaking it if desired.
5. Add a slice of provolone, half a slice of grated Swiss cheese, and one tablespoon of Parmesan cheese to the top of each piece of bread.
6. After placing the dish on a cookie sheet, bake it in the preheated oven for two to three minutes, or until the cheese is bubbling and starting to brown.
7. Enjoy while hot!

MY OBSERVATIONS

Roasted Root Vegetables

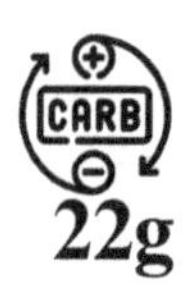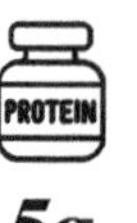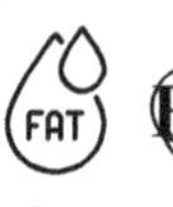

Prep	Cook	CARB	KCAL	PROTEIN	FAT	Fibre	Servings
30 mins	47 mins	22g	144 Cal	5g	3g	4.1g	6

Ingredients

- 1 cup chopped raw beets
- 4 carrots, finely chopped
- 1 finely chopped onion
- 2 cups chopped potatoes
- 4 cloves of garlic, minced
- ¼ cup canned chickpeas, drained
- 2 tablespoons of olive oil
- 1 tablespoon dried thyme leaves
- salt and pepper to taste
- ⅓ cup dry white wine
- 1 cup grated beet greens

Instructions

1. Oven temperature should be set to 400 F, or 200 C. In a 9 x 13-inch baking dish, combine the beets, carrots, onions, potatoes, garlic, and chickpeas.

2. Add a drizzle of olive oil and season with salt, pepper, and thyme. Blend thoroughly.

3. Put in the oven that has been preheated, uncovered, and bake for thirty minutes, stirring once. After taking the dish out of the oven, stir in the wine. Put it back in the oven and continue cooking for another 15 minutes or so, or until the wine has mostly evaporated and the vegetables are soft.

4. Add the beet greens and allow the heat from the leaves to cause them to wilt. Add salt and pepper to the preferred taste before you start to eat.

MY OBSERVATIONS

Slow Cooker Dahl

  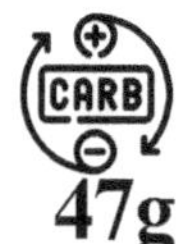 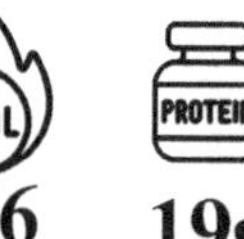 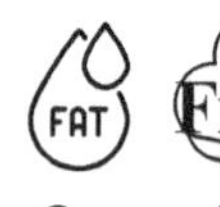 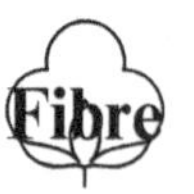 

Prep	Cook	CARB	KCAL	PROTEIN	FAT	Fibre	Servings
25 mins	55+ mins	47g	356 Cal	19g	9g	7.1g	4

Ingredients

- 300 g / 10 ½ oz yellow split peas
- 1 chopped onion
- 200 g chopped tomatoes (canned or fresh)
- Finely chopped fresh ginger root
- 2 teaspoons of cumin seeds, 1 teaspoon crushed in a mortar
- 2 teaspoons of turmeric powder
- 2 cloves of garlic, one crushed and one thin slice
- 10 freeze-dried curry leaves
- 700 ml / 1¼ point hot vegetable stock
- 1 red pepper, thinly sliced
- 2 tablespoons of vegetable or sunflower oil
- Lemon wedges, to serve

Instructions

1. Stir in the split peas, onions, tomatoes, curry leaves, minced garlic, ginger, cumin powder, turmeric, and broth in the slow cooker.

2. Stir in most of the peppers. Once the peas are tender, cook for 4 hours. Add plenty of freshly ground black pepper and salt to the dal to taste. Warm up the oil in a saucepan right before serving. Diced garlic and whole cumin seeds should be added when the oil is very hot. The cumin should start to taste roasted and almost smoky as the garlic turns golden.

3. Add some more green chilies, drizzle hot seasoned oil over the Dahl, and serve with lemon wedges drizzled over.

MY OBSERVATIONS

Slow Cooker Oats

  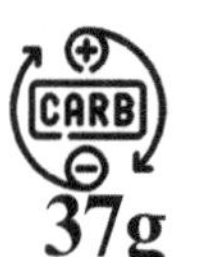  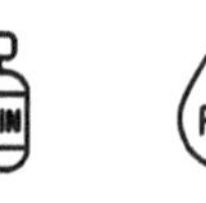 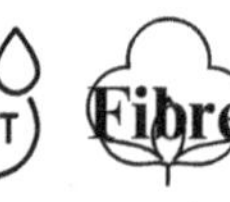 

Prep	Cook	CARB	KCAL	PROTEIN	FAT	Fibre	Servings
10 mins	310 mins	37g	208 Cal	4g	6g	4g	6

Ingredients

- 3 ½ cups water
- 1 cup steel-cut oats (steel-cut only)
- 1 cup peeled and chopped apples
- ½ cup raisins
- 2 tablespoons of butter
- 2 tablespoons of brown sugar
- 1 teaspoon of vanilla extract

Instructions

1. In a slow cooker, combine water, vanilla, raisins, oats, brown sugar, butter, and apples. Mix thoroughly until the sugar is completely dissolved.
2. Cook the oats covered over low heat for 6 to 7 hours, or until they are soft and creamy. Cook 8 hours to get the desired texture.
3. Cook on warm instead of low heat if your slow cooker becomes too hot to handle.

MY OBSERVATIONS

Leek Fritter

  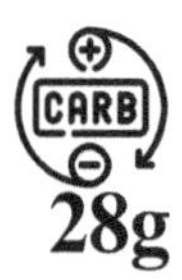  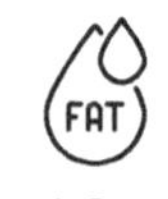 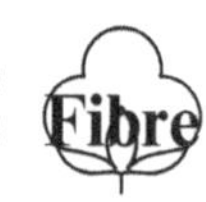 

Prep	Cook	CARB	KCAL	PROTEIN	FAT	Fibre	Servings
10 mins	15 mins	28g	335 Cal	13.3g	18g	4g	6

Ingredients

- 2 tablespoons of unsalted butter and 1 nut
- 2 washed leeks, halved lengthwise and thinly sliced
- 3 gardens
- 200 g self-rising flour
- 100 g finely grated aged cheddar
- 1 tablespoon whole grain mustard
- 75 ml
- Salad
- 1 long shallot, finely chopped
- 2 tablespoons of red wine vinegar
- 1 cup Dijon mustard
- 2 tablespoons of extra virgin olive oil
- 90 grams of water
- Small bunch of flat-leaf parsley, leaves torn off

Instructions

1. 1.In a nonstick skillet, melt the butter over low heat while carefully sautéing the leeks for ten minutes, or until they are soft, adding a dash of salt.
2. Transfer it to a big bowl and allow it to cool.
3. Combine the eggs, flour, mustard, cheddar, and seasoning; gradually whisk in the milk until the mixture reaches a thick consistency
4. Assemble the salad and transfer the mustard, vinegar, oil, and a small amount of seasoning into a different bowl.
5. In a nonstick pan, melt a knob of butter and add two to three tablespoons of dough. Cook for two to three minutes, or until golden brown, then turn and continue.
6. To enjoy the remaining donuts (you should have about a dozen),

arrange the cooked ones on a baking tray and reheat them in a low oven.

7. Just before serving, thoroughly combine the vinaigrette with the watercress and parsley. Spoon the fried leeks onto individual plates and accompany with the salad.

MY OBSERVATIONS

Mozzarella Sticks With Spicy Dipping

 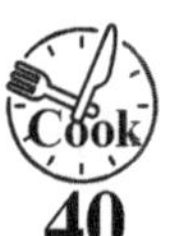 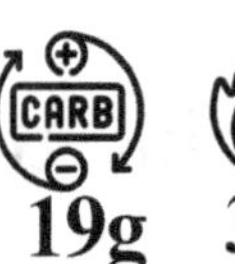 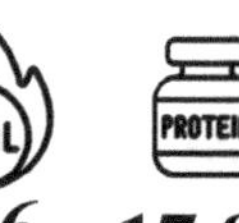 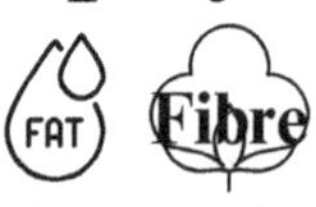 

Prep	Cook	CARB	KCAL	PROTEIN	FAT	Fibre	Servings
15 mins	40 mins	19g	386 Cal	17.8g	25.6g	1.7g	6

Ingredients

- 400g mozzarella
- 3 tablespoons coarsely seasoned white flour
- 2 eggs, beaten and prepared
- 100g panko breadcrumbs
- 1 teaspoon garlic salt
- 1 teaspoon dried oregano
- Oil for deep frying
- Sauce
- 1 ½ tablespoons olive oil
- 1 tablespoon of butter
- ½ chopped onion
- 1 clove of garlic, minced
- Dry red pepper flakes, a good pinch
- ¼ teaspoon smoked paprika
- 100 g canned crushed tomatoes

Instructions

1. 1.Slice the mozzarella thickly, then cut each slice into 2 cm wide fingers. Set aside to rest for 10 minutes on paper towels.

2. In a separate bowl, combine the panko, flour, and egg. Mix the oregano and garlic salt into the breadcrumbs. Place parchment paper inside a baking dish. Start by dipping the mozzarella sticks into the flour mixture, followed by the eggs and breadcrumbs. After layering, place the layers in a bowl and freeze. After freezing, move to a freezer.

3. Before preparing the fish, preheat the butter and olive oil in a pan and sauté the onion and garlic until they are tender. Simmer the tomatoes, sugar, paprika, and chilli flakes for 15 minutes, or until the mixture thickens. Hold until firm and smooth with a stick. Before eating, thaw it in a

saucepan if needed, and boil it for five minutes.

4. Heat the pan to 180°C or until the bread browns in 30 seconds after adding ⅓ of oil to it. Straight out of the freezer, fry the mozzarella sticks for 4–5 minutes, or until golden brown. Then, drain them on a baking sheet. Accompany with a warm dip.

MY OBSERVATIONS

This page was intentionally left blank.

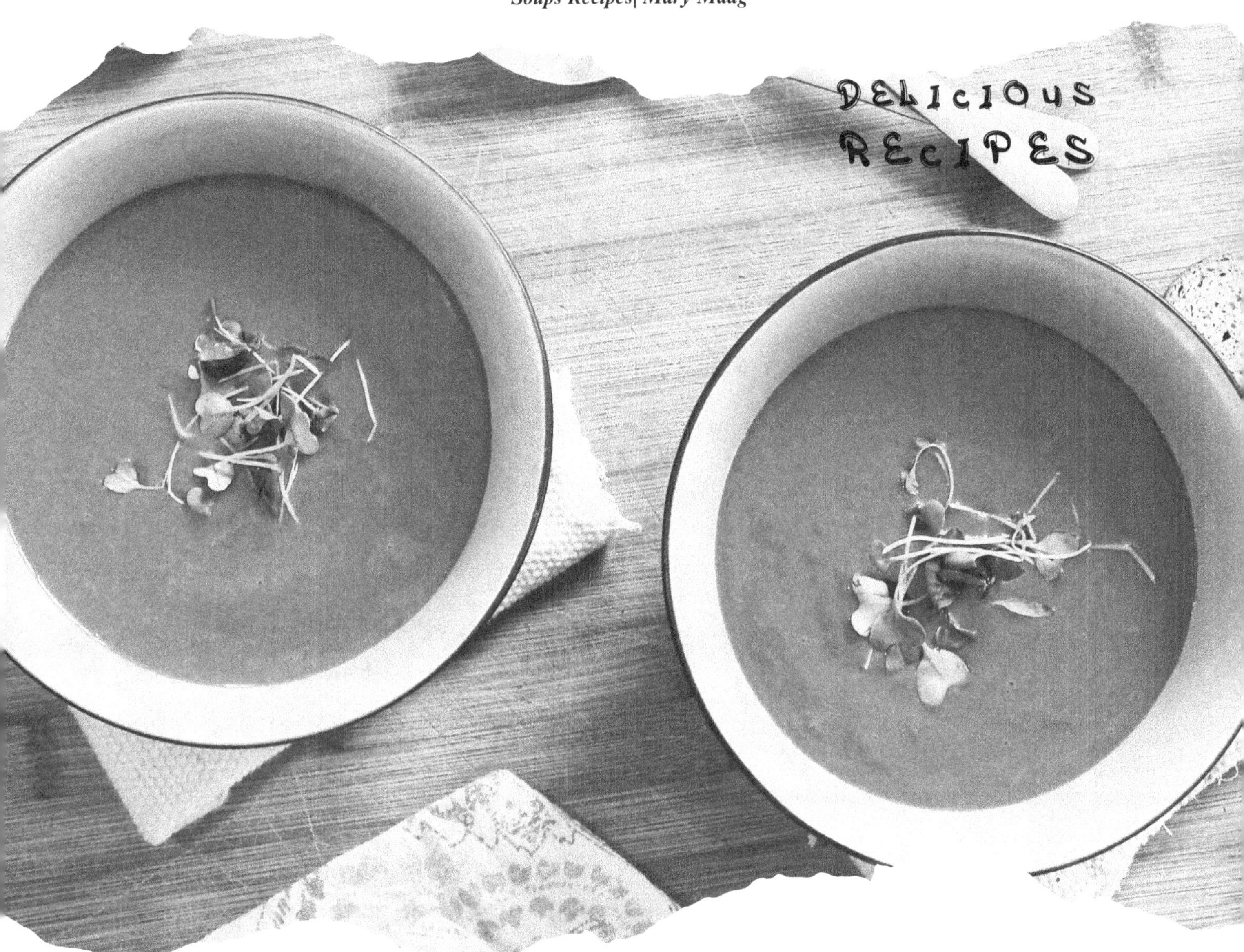

SOUPS
RECIPES

—— FOR HEALTHY YOU ——

Tomato Basil soup

  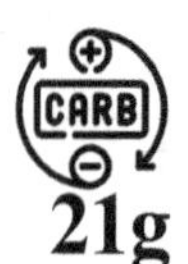  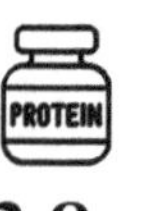 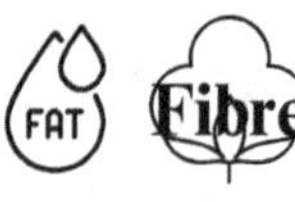 

Prep	Cook	CARB	KCAL	PROTEIN	FAT	Fibre	Servings
15 mins	90 mins	21g	214 Cal	3.8g	13.2g	3.4g	8

Ingredients

- ¼ cup extra-virgin olive oil, divided
- 1 teaspoon thyme leaves
- 1 tablespoon balsamic vinegar
- 2½ pounds roma tomatoes, halved
- 1 loose-packed cup basil leaves, more for garnish
- 1 medium yellow onion, chopped
- Sea salt and freshly ground black pepper
- ⅓ cup chopped carrots
- 3 cups vegetable broth
  4 garlic cloves, chopped

Instructions

1. Adjust the oven temperature to 350°F and place parchment paper on a large baking sheet. On the baking sheet, arrange the tomatoes cut-side up. Drizzle with two tablespoons of olive oil and season with salt and pepper. Roast until the insides are still juicy and the edges are just beginning to shrivel, about 1 hour.

2. In a large pot over medium heat, warm the remaining 2 tablespoons of olive oil. Simmer the onions, carrots, garlic, and ½ teaspoon of salt for 8 minutes or until the vegetables are tender. After adding the tomatoes, vinegar, vegetable broth, and thyme leaves, simmer for 20 minutes.

3. Once the soup has cooled down a little, transfer it to a blender, blending it in batches if needed. Mix until it looks homogenous. Pulse to join the basil.

4. Serve with bread and basil leaf.

MY OBSERVATIONS

Parsnip Soup

  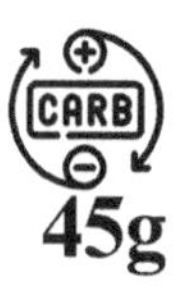 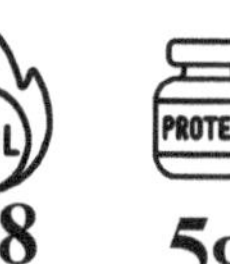 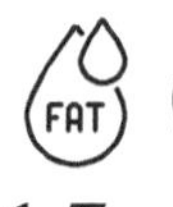 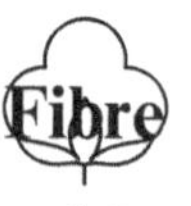 

Prep	Cook	CARB	KCAL	PROTEIN	FAT	Fibre	Servings
20 mins	20 mins	45g	198 Cal	5g	1.7g	10g	4

Ingredients

- 1/2 tsp Dried chilli flakes
- 2 Cloves garlic
- 300 ml Milk
- 800g Parsnips
- 1 Onion
- 750 ml Stock
- Salt and freshly ground black pepper
- 4 tbsp Olive oil
- 2 tbsp Parmesan cheese
- Extra virgin olive oil
- 300 g Cubes of bread

Instructions

1. In a large saucepan, combine the parsnips, onion, garlic, chilli flakes, stock, salt, and pepper.
2. Cook until the parsnips are very tender, about 20 minutes over medium heat.
3. Blend in the milk until smooth.
4. Set oven temperature to 200°C.
5. Mix the oil, garlic, Parmesan, salt, and pepper with the bread cubes.
6. Arrange the cubes in a single layer on a baking sheet, leaving ample space between them, and bake for approximately ten minutes. (Watch them carefully because they can burn.)

MY OBSERVATIONS

Turkey Chili

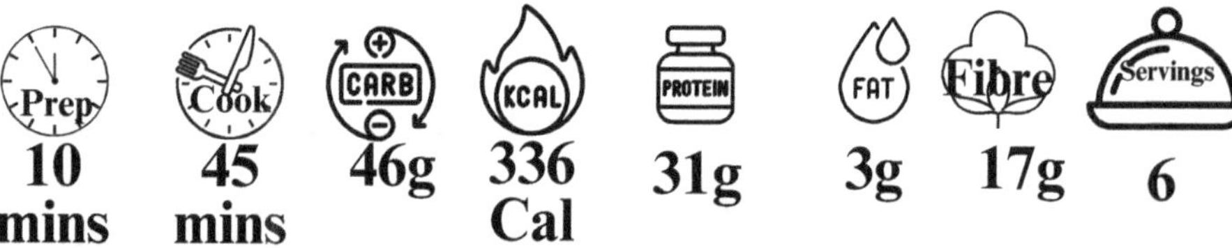

Ingredients

- 1 1/4 cup chicken broth and 3 minced garlic cloves
- 2 tsp ground cumin
- 1 1/4 teaspoon of cayenne
- 2 tsp olive oil
- 3 minced garlic cloves
- 1 pound of extra-lean ground chicken or turkey
- 1 can of diced or crushed tomatoes
- 1 can of rinsed and drained sweet corn
- 1 1/2 teaspoon salt and additional to taste
- 2 cans of rinsed and drained dark red kidney beans
- 4 tsp of chili powder
- 1 tsp of dehydrated oregano
- 1 chopped yellow onion
- 1 chopped medium red bell pepper

Instructions

1. Fill a big pot with oil and heat it to a medium-high temperature. Stirring constantly, sauté the onion, garlic, and red pepper for five to seven minutes.

2. Break up the meat and add the ground turkey. Cook until the meat is no longer pink. Add the salt, cayenne pepper, oregano, cumin, chili powder, and stir for about 20 seconds.

3. Corn, kidney beans, tomatoes, and chicken broth should then be added. Once the chili thickens and the flavors meld, bring it to a boil, then lower the heat and simmer it for 30 to 45 minutes. Taste and adjust salt and seasonings accordingly.

4. Add any kind of garnish that you like.

MY OBSERVATIONS

Quinoa Herbed soup

  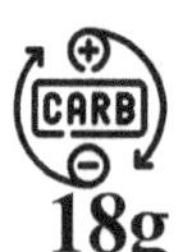  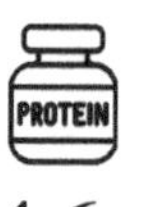 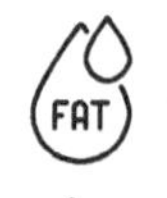 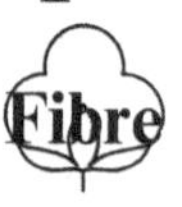 

Prep	Cook	CARB	KCAL	PROTEIN	FAT	Fibre	Servings
15 mins	30 mins	18g	126 Cal	4.6g	4g	4.2g	6

Ingredients

- 1 1/2 tablespoons of pure virgin olive oil
- 1 1/2 large onions, minced garlic cloves, chopped, and 2 cups of carrot slices
- 8 ounces of sliced white button mushrooms, 2 cups of sliced celery, and 2 teaspoons of dried basil
- 1 tsp crushed dried rosemary leaves
- 1½ teaspoon of dried thyme
- 1/2 tsp freshly ground black pepper
- Rinse 1/2 cup of quinoa and 64 ounces of veggie broth.
- Swiss chard leaves, chopped; 4 cups

Instructions

1. Heat oil in a big pot or Dutch oven over medium heat. Saute the onion, garlic, carrots, celery, mushrooms, herbs, and pepper for approximately ten minutes, or until the onions and mushrooms become tender.

2. When the quinoa and broth are combined, bring to a boil, then lower the heat and simmer for 15 minutes, or until the carrots and quinoa are soft.

3. Swiss chard should be boiled for three minutes, or until it is tender, in a large pot of water. Empty the. Add the chard to the soup. Turn over.

MY OBSERVATIONS

Spicy Collards

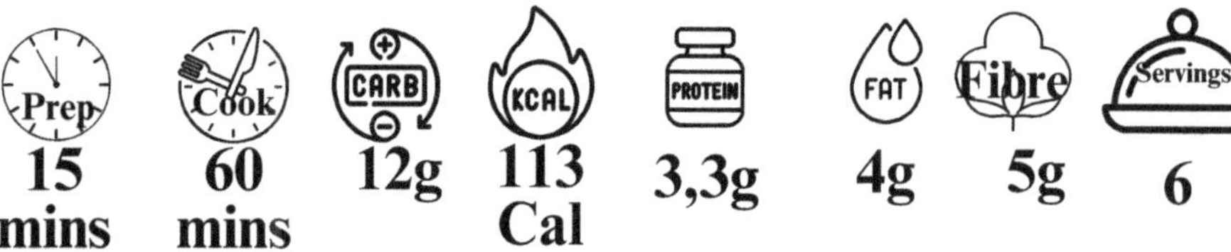

Prep	Cook	CARB	KCAL	PROTEIN	FAT	Fibre	Servings
15 mins	60 mins	12g	113 Cal	3,3g	4g	5g	6

Ingredients

- 2 pounds of rinsed collard greens
- 5 slices of diced bacon
- 1 big onion, chopped
- 3 tablespoons of cider vinegar and 3/4 cup of chicken broth
- 1 tablespoon of sugar, dark brown
- 1 tsp red pepper flakes
- 1/4 to 1/2 tspn hot sauce, such as Tabasco sauce
- Pepper and salt

Instructions

1. For each collard green leaf, make a cut with a knife on both sides of the large rib. Take it off and throw it away. Scoop out the thickest portion of the leaf; no need to cut all the way up. Just cut off the stem if the leaf is smaller. To make 1/2-inch strips, stack four to five leaves, roll them up, and cut. Repeat with the remaining foliage.

2. Crisp up bacon by cooking it in a big pot over medium heat. Transfer to a dish covered with paper towels using a slotted spoon.

3. Stir onion until softened while cooking over medium heat in bacon fat, stirring occasionally.

4. Transfer the broth, vinegar, sugar, Tabasco sauce, and red pepper flakes into the pot. Toss to mix.

MY OBSERVATIONS

Brussels soup

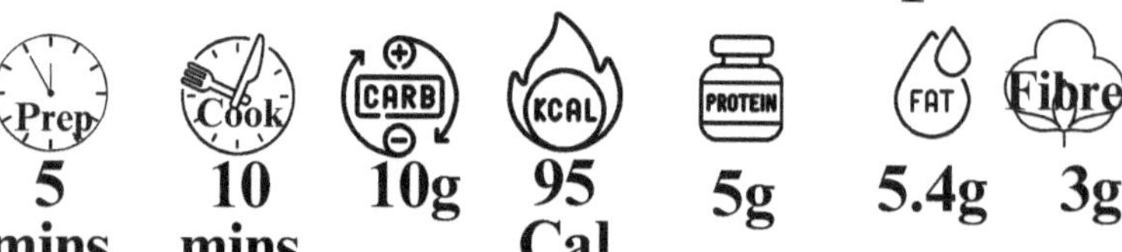

Ingredients

- 350 grams, or 12.35 ounces Trimmed Brussels sprouts, ½ cup (100 g) in weight small pieces (3.53 oz) frozen
- 1 finely chopped onion
- 1 or two finely chopped garlic cloves
- 1 tablespoon of olive oil
- 2 tsp butter for every three cups (700 ml) vegetable broth
- Black or white pepper to taste

Instructions

1. Cut off the ends of the Brussels sprouts and remove any loose leaves. Rinse and weigh the sprouts.
2. Add to a blender and pulse to shred finely.
3. Heat the oil in a medium-sized pot, add the onion and garlic, and cook over medium heat for 3–4 minutes, stirring frequently, until softened.
4. Stir in the chopped Brussels sprouts and cook for an additional minute.
5. After adding the stock and seasoning with pepper, cover and bring to a boil. After five minutes, reduce the heat and simmer.
6. To fully reheat, add the petits pois and cook for an additional minute.
7. Take the soup off the stove and puree it. Serve after adding the butter and adjusting the seasoning to taste.

MY OBSERVATIONS

Turkey and Kale Soup

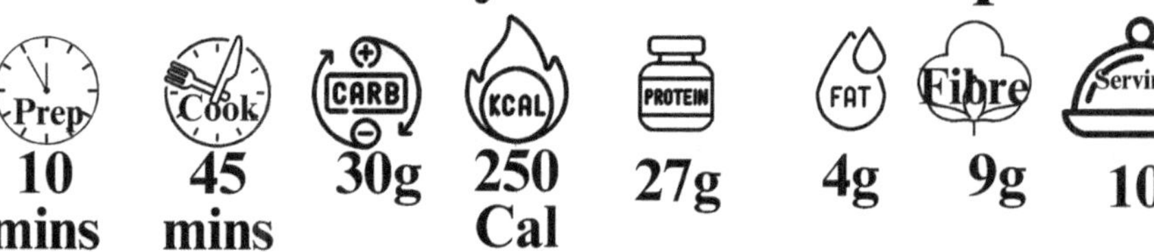

Prep	Cook	CARB	KCAL	PROTEIN	FAT	Fibre	Servings
10 mins	45 mins	30g	250 Cal	27g	4g	9g	10

Ingredients

- 5 cups Remove and chop the stems from the kale.
- 1/2 pound of ground turkey
- 1 cup of reduced-sodium vegetable broth
- 1 cup of rinsed and dried lima beans
- 1 cup of rinsed and dried white beans
- 6 cups of water
- Tomatoes, chopped, without salt
- 1/2 minced onion
- 2 tufts Diced celery, onion, and two carrots
- 1 teaspoon each of pepper and salt, adjusted to taste
- 1.5 tablespoons oregano
- 5 tablespoons of basil
- 1 tablespoon of extra virgin olive oil

Instructions

1. Once the beans are soft but not mushy, cook them with water under high pressure for about 30 minutes.
2. Drain the beans after taking them out of the instant pot.
3. In the instant pot, sauté the onion, carrots, garlic, and celery in a tablespoon of olive oil until the vegetables are fragrant. Keep the cover on.
4. When the turkey has browned, add the ground turkey and sauté.
5. As much kale as possible should be added to the pot along with the remaining ingredients.
6. You can now shut the lid and cook for about three minutes on high pressure.
7. Enjoy.

MY OBSERVATIONS

Pumpkin soup

  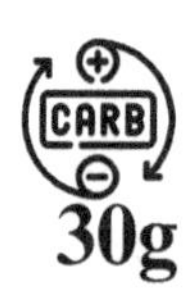  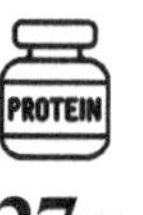 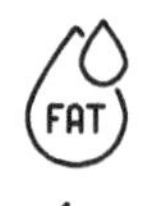 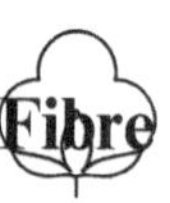 

Prep	Cook	CARB	KCAL	PROTEIN	FAT	Fibre	Servings
10 mins	45 mins	30g	250 Cal	27g	4g	9g	8

Ingredients

- 1.2 kg / 2.4 lb unpeeled butternut squash OR pumpkin (any variety) (Note 1)
- 1 sliced onion (yellow, brown, or white)
- 2 whole peeled garlic cloves
- 3 cups low-sodium vegetable or chicken broth or stock
- one cup of water
- Add pepper and salt.

Instructions

1. Slice the pumpkin into rounds that are 3cm/2.25 in. Slice off the skin and remove the seeds with a spoon (a video helps). Cut into pieces that are 4 cm/1.5".

2. The liquid in the pot won't completely submerge the pumpkin, so add the onion, garlic, broth, and water. Bring to a boil, uncovered, then lower heat and quickly simmer for about ten minutes, or until pumpkin is tender when tested with a butter knife.

3. Take off the stove and blend with a stick blender (Note 3 for blender) until smooth.

4. Add salt and pepper to taste, then stir in the cream (do not boil the soup after adding the cream, as it will split).

5. Spoon soup into individual bowls, top with a little cream, and garnish with parsley and pepper, if preferred. Accompany with freshly baked bread.

MY OBSERVATIONS

Curried Okra soup

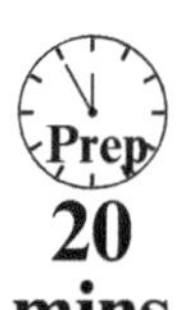  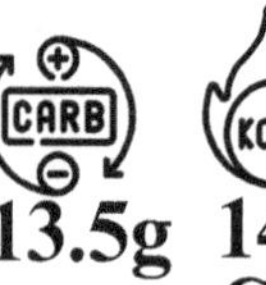 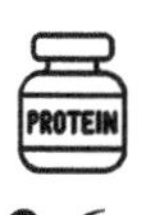 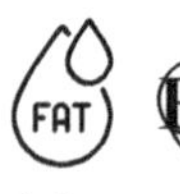 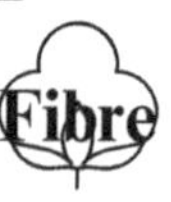 

Prep	Cook	CARB	KCAL	PROTEIN	FAT	Fibre	Servings
20 mins	120 mins	13.5g	149 Cal	3,6g	10g	4g	6

Ingredients

- 1 pound of young okra pods
- 2 onions
- 3 tablespoons of olive oil.
- 1 1/2 teaspoon of dried, hot, red chili pepper
- 1/4 to 1/2 teaspoon of mild curry powder.
- 1/4 teaspoon of ground turmeric, plus salt and pepper to taste

Instructions

1. Trim the okra pods at the ends.
2. Cut the pods into rounds that are between 1/4 and 1/2 inch in diameter.
3. Slice and peel the onions.
4. After slicing the okra, transfer it to a glass or stainless steel bowl and generously season with salt.
5. Make sure all of the slices are submerged in the iced water when you cover them, and then chill for at least two hours.
6. Take the bowl out of the fridge and pour the salt water out of it.
7. In a heavy skillet, heat the oil over medium-high heat.
8. Saute the okra until it turns a light brown. (Roughly ten minutes).
9. Rotate regularly to avoid sticking.
10. When the onions are soft, add the remaining ingredients and continue to fry for an additional three minutes.

184

MY OBSERVATIONS

Butternut Soup

  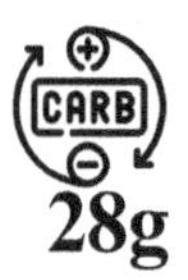  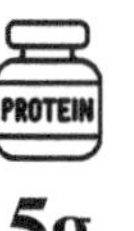 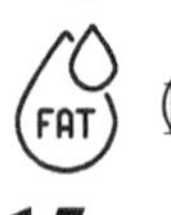 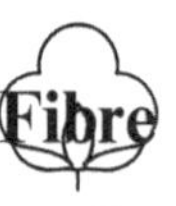 

Prep	Cook	CARB	KCAL	PROTEIN	FAT	Fibre	Servings
15 mins	50 mins	28g	264 Cal	5g	15g	6g	6

Ingredients

- 1 butternut squash (about one kilogram), deseeded and peeled
- 2 tablespoons of olive oil
- 1 tablespoon of butter
- 2 chopped onions
- 1 thinly sliced garlic clove and two mild red chilies, deseeded and chopped finely
- 850ml vegetables stock, hot
- 4 tablespoons crème fraîche, plus additional to serve

Instructions

1. Preheat the oven to 200°C (fan 180°C) and gas 6.
2. Cut the squash into large cubes that are about 4 cm/1½ inches across, and then toss it with 1 tablespoon of olive oil in a large roasting tin.
3. Roast for 30 minutes, tossing once, or until tender and golden.
4. In a large saucepan, melt the butter with the remaining tablespoon of olive oil and add the onions, garlic clove, and three-quarters of the chillies while the butternut squash cooks.
5. When the onions are very soft, cook them covered for 15 to 20 minutes over very low heat.
6. After adding the crème fraîche and stock to the pan with the butternut squash, blend everything together using a stick blender until it's smooth. If you want a really smooth soup, blend the soup in a blender.
7. Taste-test and return to the pan to reheat gently.

MY OBSERVATIONS

This page was intentionally left blank.

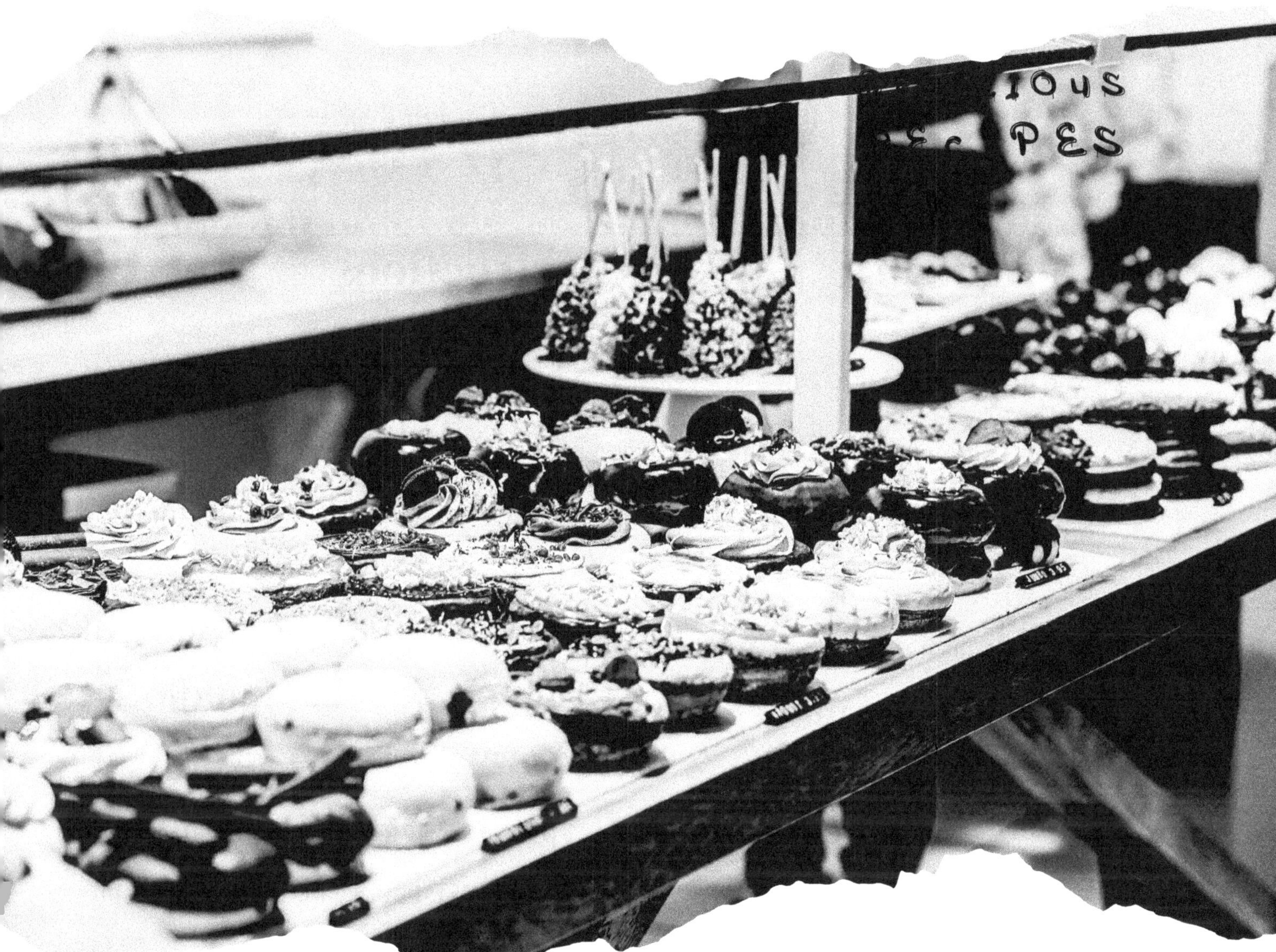

SNACKS
RECIPES

—— FOR HEALTHY YOU ——

189

Baked Grapefruits

  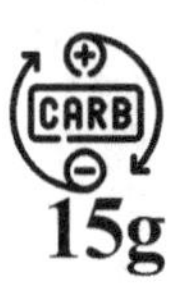 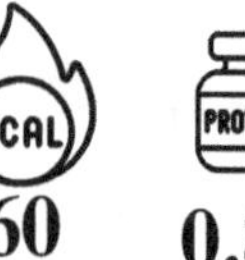 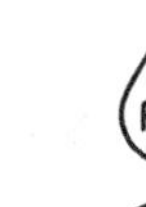 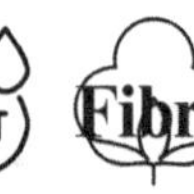 

Prep	Cook	CARB	KCAL	PROTEIN	FAT	Fibre	Servings
10 mins	15 mins	15g	60 Cal	0.8g	1g	0.5g	4

Ingredients

- 2 grapefruits
- 4 teaspoons of either clear honey or maple syrup
- 1 teaspoon of finely ground cinnamon

Instructions

1. Using a knife, cut grapefruit halves and remove the pith.
2. Let the sections slack.
3. Put a small amount of honey in the middle of every grapefruit. Alternatively, pour honey or maple syrup over the top.
4. Add a dash of cinnamon.
5. Bake for 15 minutes at 190C/375F.

MY OBSERVATIONS

Cucumber Slices with Tzatziki

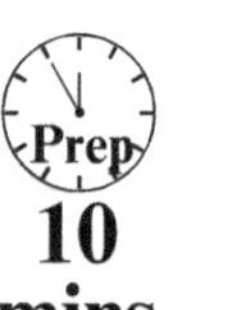  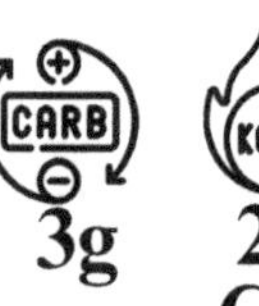 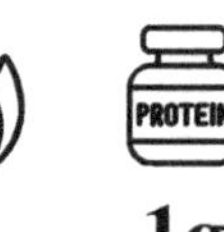 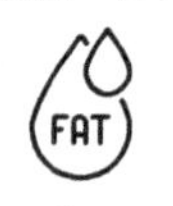 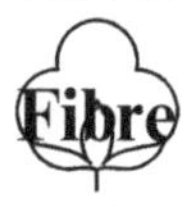 

Prep	Cook	CARB	KCAL	PROTEIN	FAT	Fibre	Servings
10 mins	00 mins	3g	27 Cal	1g	1g	1g	4

Ingredients

- 1 English Cucumber
- 1/4 tiny red onion, to taste
- A tsp of lemon juice
- Half a cup of whole-fat plain Greek yogurt
- 2-3 tablespoons finely minced fresh dill
- 10 to 20 fresh mint leaves, chopped finely
- 1 1/2 teaspoon of dry oregano
- A tsp of salt and a tsp of ground black pepper.

Instructions

1. Very thinly slice the cucumber, and chop the circles into quarters if you prefer smaller pieces. There ought to be roughly two cups of cucumber chopped.
2. Cut the red onion into thin slices, then roughly chop the slices to match the size of your cucumber pieces. Sliced red onion, lemon juice, and salt should be combined in a small, non-reactive bowl (such as a glass, stainless steel, or ceramic bowl); stir, then set aside while you gather the remaining ingredients.
3. Cucumber, red onion, lemon juice, and the remaining ingredients should all be combined in a big bowl. Mix thoroughly. If necessary, adjust the flavor by adding more lemon juice or salt.
4. Savor it right away or put it in the fridge to consume it in a day or two.

192

MY OBSERVATIONS

Mozzarella marinade

  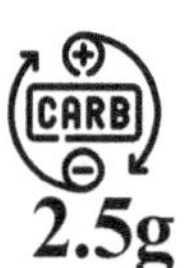  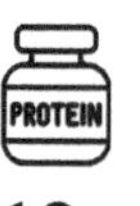 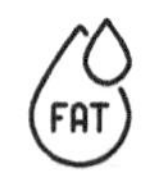 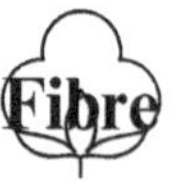 

Prep	Cook	CARB	KCAL	PROTEIN	FAT	Fibre	Servings
15 mins	00 mins	2.5g	204 Cal	12g	16g	0.1g	10

Ingredients

- 1/3 cup extra virgin olive oil
- 1 tablespoon of chopped, oil-rich sun-dried tomatoes
- 1 tablespoon of freshly chopped parsley
- 1 tablespoon finely chopped red pepper flakes
- 1 tablespoon of dried basil
- 1 teaspoon finely chopped chives
- 1/4 teaspoon powdered garlic
- Cubed part-skim mozzarella cheese, 1 pound

Instructions

1. Mix the first seven ingredients in a big bowl and then add the cheese cubes. To coat, stir. Cover and chill for a minimum of half an hour.

MY OBSERVATIONS

Healthy pizza

  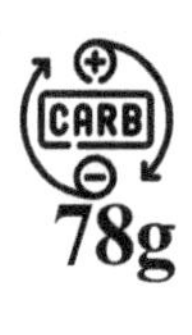  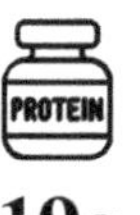 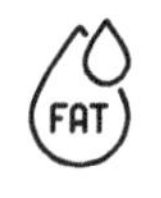 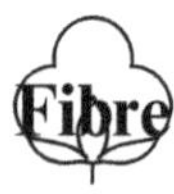 

Prep	Cook	CARB	KCAL	PROTEIN	FAT	Fibre	Servings
15 mins	12 mins	78g	479 Cal	19g	13g	10g	2

Ingredients

- 100g of each robust wholewheat and white flour
- 1 teaspoon or seven grams of easy-blend dried yeast sachet
- 125milliliters of warm water.
- To make the topping, chop 200g of tomato, squeeze out the juice, finely chop a handful of cherry tomatoes, and cut one large courgette in half and thinly slice it with a peeler.
- 25 grams of shredded mozzarella
- 1 tablespoon of brined capers, drained; eight green olives, coarsely chopped
- 1 finely chopped garlic clove
- A tablespoon of olive oil
- To serve, add 2 tablespoons of chopped parsley.

Instructions

1. In a food processor fitted with a dough blade, combine the flours, yeast, and a small pinch of salt. After adding the water and mixing to form a soft dough, work for one minute. Once the dough is removed, roll it out to a round shape about 30 cm across on a surface dusted with flour. Transfer to a baking sheet coated with oil.

2. Cover the dough with the canned tomatoes, leaving a 2-centimeter border around it. Sprinkle the mozzarella on top after arranging the cherry tomatoes and courgettes on top. Stir together the garlic, olives, and capers, then sprinkle on top. Distribute the oil evenly. Give it 20 minutes to rise. Preheat the oven to 240°C, 220°F for the fan, gas 9, or the highest setting.

3. Pizza should be baked for 10 to 12 minutes, or until the edges are crisp and golden. Finally, garnish with parsley and serve.

MY OBSERVATIONS

Rice cake

  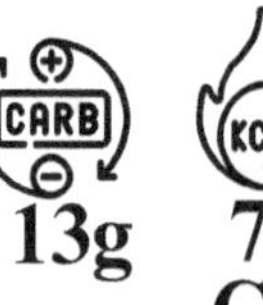 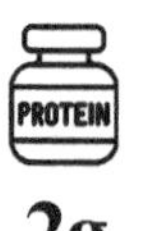 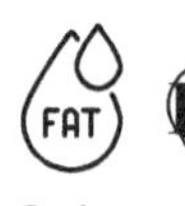 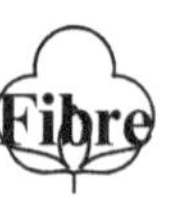 

Prep	Cook	CARB	KCAL	PROTEIN	FAT	Fibre	Servings
2 mins	45 mins	13g	73 Cal	2g	24g	1g	2

Ingredients

- 1 cup of raw rice
- 1 1/2 cup of water
- 2 eggs
- 2 tablespoons of all-purpose flour.
- Flavors for gluten-free flour: Use 1 teaspoon each of salt, pepper, and 2 teaspoons of parmesan cheese for savory.
- To make sweets, use 1 teaspoon of cinnamon and 2-3 Truvia envelopes.

Instructions

1. Set oven temperature to 350 degrees Fahrenheit.
2. Grind the raw rice in a food processor or blender until it's finely ground.
3. Add the remaining ingredients to a food processor or blender set on high speed.
4. Transfer the batter into a muffin tin, donut pan, or any other shaped pan that has been greased (silicone does not require frying).
5. Bake for 40 to 50 minutes, or until crispy on all sides and the tops are browned.

MY OBSERVATIONS

Carrot Sticks with Hummus

  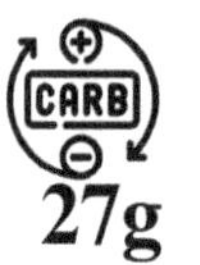 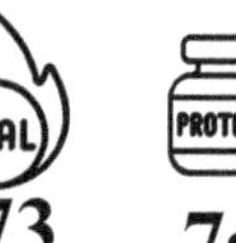 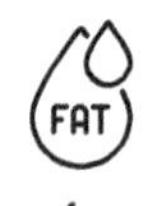 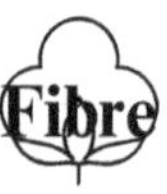 

Prep	Cook	CARB	KCAL	PROTEIN	FAT	Fibre	Servings
5 mins	10 mins	27g	173 Cal	7g	4g	8g	6

Ingredients

- 15 oz (400 g) of chickpeas, 1 can (drained), and ¼ cup (60 mL) of olive oil
- Juiced half lemon
- 1 tiny garlic clove
- ¼ teaspoon of cumin powder
- Kosher salt
- 6 medium-sized carrots

Instructions

1. In a blender or food processor, combine the chickpeas, olive oil, lemon juice, garlic, cumin, and salt; process until fully smooth.
2. Transfer to an airtight jar and keep in the refrigerator for a maximum of seven days.
3. Slice and peel the carrots to make spears.
4. Accompany with ⅓ cup (80 g) of hummus.
5. Enjoy!

MY OBSERVATIONS

Apple Chips

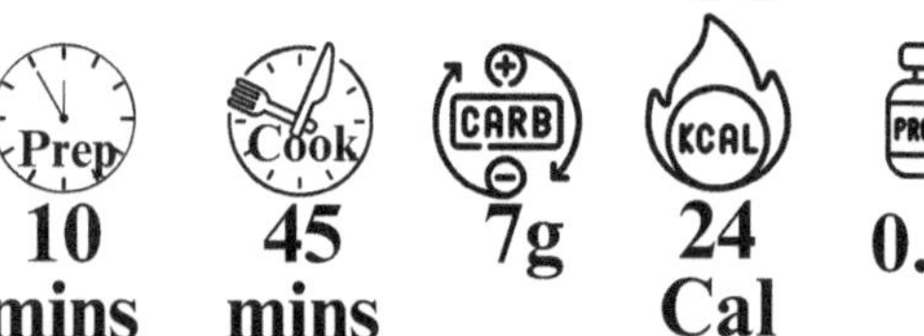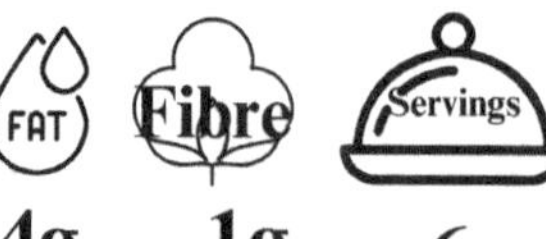

Prep	Cook	CARB	KCAL	PROTEIN	FAT	Fibre	Servings
10 mins	45 mins	7g	24 Cal	0.1g	4g	1g	6

Ingredients

- 1/2 tsp white sugar
- One-half teaspoon of ground cinnamon
- 2 cored and thinly sliced Golden Delicious apples

Instructions

1. Set the oven's temperature to 225°F, or 110°C. Put parchment paper on one side of a metal baking sheet.
2. Place apple slices on the prepared baking sheet in a single layer.
3. In a small bowl, combine sugar and cinnamon; sprinkle over apple slices.
4. Bake for 45 to 1 hour, or until the apples are dried out and the edges begin to curl, in a preheated oven. Chips should be cooled and crisped before being moved to a wire rack using a metal spatula.

MY OBSERVATIONS

Apple Pie

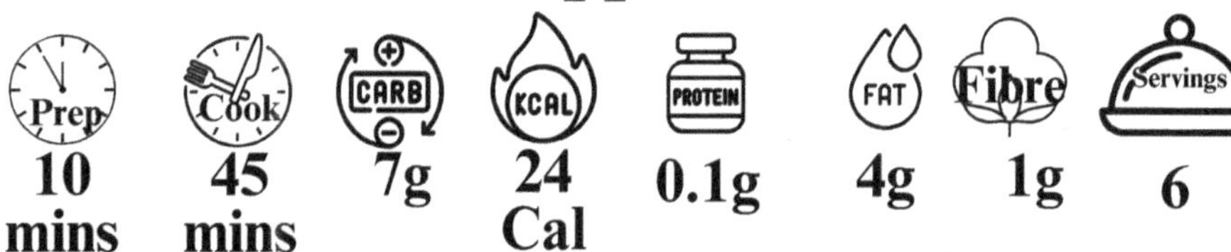

Prep	Cook	CARB	KCAL	PROTEIN	FAT	Fibre	Servings
10 mins	45 mins	7g	24 Cal	0.1g	4g	1g	6

Ingredients

- 8 tiny green apples, or more as necessary
- One-half cup unsalted butter
- Three tsp of all-purpose flour
- One-half cup of white sugar
- Half a cup of dense brown sugar
- A quarter cup of water
- One nine-inch pie crust, thawed from the freezer

Instructions

1. After peeling and cored, thinly slice the apples. Put aside.
2. Bake at 425 degrees Fahrenheit (220 degrees Celsius).
3. In a medium heat saucepan, melt the butter. Cook for one to two minutes, or until fragrant, after adding flour and stirring to make a paste. Bring the water to a boil after adding the sugars. Simmer for three to five minutes on low heat. Take off the heat source.
4. Line a 9-inch pie pan with one pastry, pressing it into the bottom and up the sides. Roll out the remaining pastry to leave about a 1/2-inch overhang on the pie. Make eight 1-inch strips out of the pastry.

5. Make a small mound with the sliced apples in the bottom crust. Using longer strips in the middle and shorter strips at the edges, arrange four pastry strips vertically and evenly spaced over the apples.

6. Create a lattice crust by completely folding the first and third strips back until they nearly hang off the pie. Unfold the first and third strips to their initial positions after placing one of the unused strips over the second and fourth strips perpendicularly.

7. The second and fourth vertical strips should be folded back. Place a perpendicularly positioned unused strip on top. Return the second and fourth strips to their initial positions by unfolding them.

8. To weave in the remaining two pastry strips, repeat Steps 6 and 7. Fold and trim any excess dough at the edges, pinching it in place.

9. Brush some of the mixture onto the lattice without letting it run off the sides. Pour the sugar-butter mixture over the lattice crust slowly and gently, making sure it seeps over the sliced apples.

10. Bake for 15 minutes in the preheated oven, then lower the temperature to 350 degrees F (175 degrees C) and bake for an additional 35 to 45 minutes, or until the apples are tender.

MY OBSERVATIONS

Almond Butter and Apple Slices

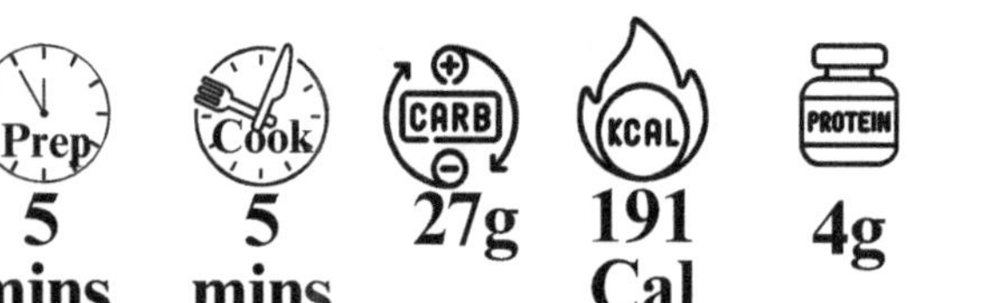

Prep	Cook	CARB	KCAL	PROTEIN	FAT	Fibre	Servings
5 mins	5 mins	27g	191 Cal	4g	9g	6g	2

Ingredients

- 2 medium size apple
- 2 tablespoon of smooth almond butter
- Ground cinnamon

Instructions

1. After cored, cut apple into 15 slices.
2. After applying a small amount of almond butter to each slice, sprinkle with cinnamon.

Seaweed Snacks

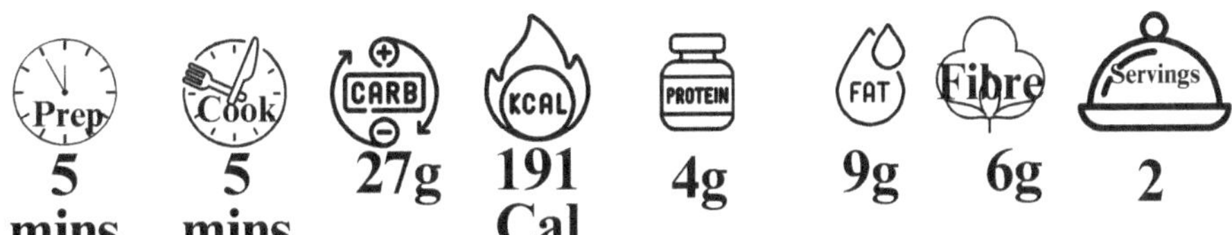

Prep	Cook	CARB	KCAL	PROTEIN	FAT	Fibre	Servings
5 mins	5 mins	27g	191 Cal	4g	9g	6g	2

Ingredients

- 5 Roasted Seaweed
- 5 sheets of Rice paper
- 1 cup olive oil or any neutral-tasting oil
- Water to moisten rice paper
- 2 teaspoon Salt
- 2 teaspoons of garlic powder
- 2 teaspoons toasted sesame seeds

Instructions

1. Place a sheet of seaweed that has been roasted rough side up. Sprinkle sesame seeds, salt, and garlic powder evenly over the seaweed.

2. Rice paper should be briefly soaked in warm water before being removed (do not soak it too long). Scatter it quickly over the sheet of roasted seaweed. Till the rice paper adheres to the seaweed, apply pressure. Fold the sides of the hanging rice paper and the corners of the empty seaweed inward.

3. While working on other pieces, transfer to a cooling rack to dry.

4. It will take some time for the rice paper to dry until it is no longer sticky to the touch. .

5. Cut each sheet into triangles of the same size with clean kitchen scissors.

6. Add the vegetable oil over medium heat, and once it's hot, use a wooden chopstick to check for bubbles. Rice paper side down, deep fry the triangles for 10 to 15 seconds, or until they are crispy, white, and slightly golden brown. It will taste burnt if you over-fry it until it is dark brown.

7. Drain extra oil from the chips. Excess oil will result in soggy chips,transfer them to a cooling rack.

MY OBSERVATIONS

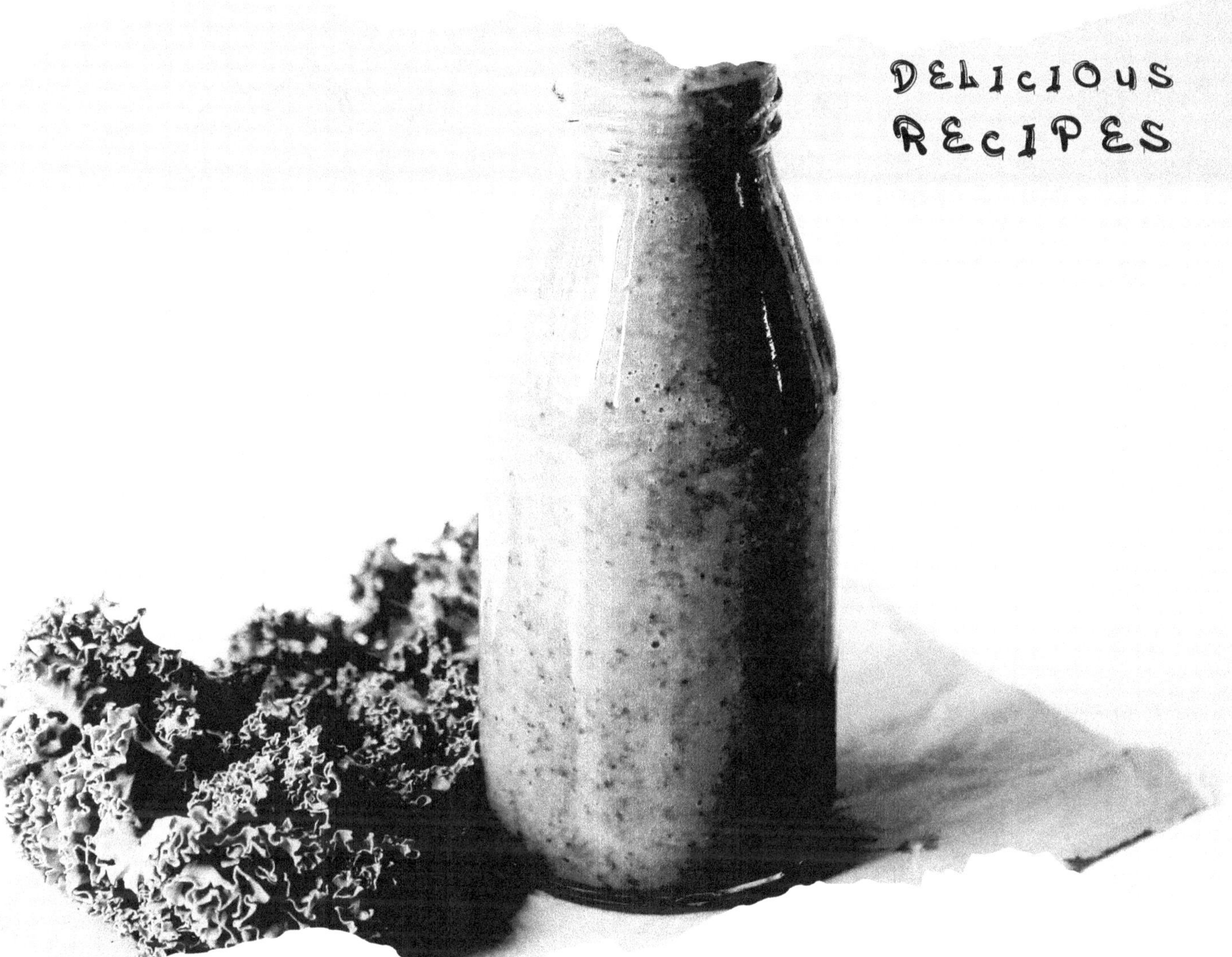

SMOOTHIES
RECIPES

—— FOR HEALTHY YOU——

Cherry Almond Smoothie

 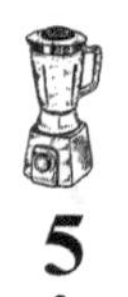 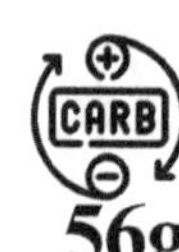  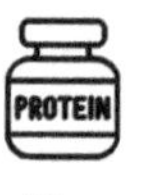 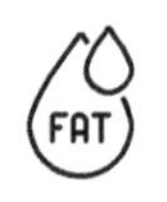 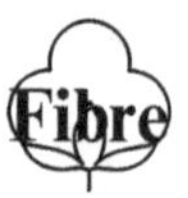 

Prep		CARB	KCAL	PROTEIN	FAT	Fibre	Servings
5 mins	5 mins	56g	326 Cal	7g	10g	11g	1

Ingredients

- 1 cup frozen cherry and berry mix
- 1 ripe banana, preferably frozen
- 2 cups organic spinach
- 1/4 teaspoon almond extract
- 1 teaspoon vanilla extract
- 1/2 cup almond milk
- 1 tablespoon almond butter
- 1 tablespoon cocoa or cacao powder(Optional)

Instructions

1. Put all the ingredients into a high-powered blender and blend until everything is creamy, smooth and looking yum yum. add more milk if you like

Banana Almond Smoothie

 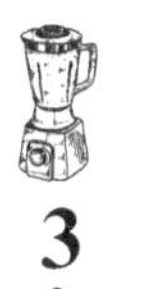 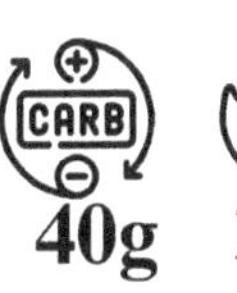 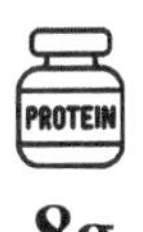 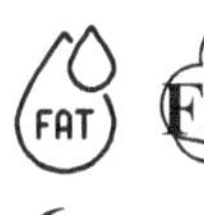 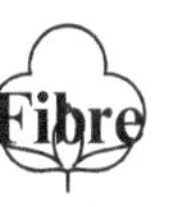 

Prep		CARB	KCAL	PROTEIN	FAT	Fibre	Servings
5 mins	3 mins	40g	213 Cal	8g	6g	4g	1

Ingredients

- 2 medium-to-large frozen banana
- ½ cup almond milk
- 2 tablespoons flax seed
- 2 teaspoon almond extract to taste.

Instructions

1. Toss all the ingredients into a blender.
2. Blend on low until the blender gains traction, then ramp up to the highest speed as soon as possible .
3. Add more maple syrup, or for more prominent almond flavor, add up to ⅛ teaspoon more almond extract, then blend again.

Tropical Paradise Smoothie

 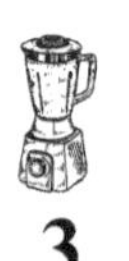 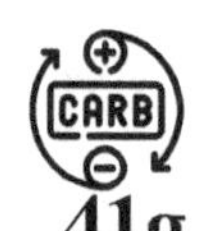  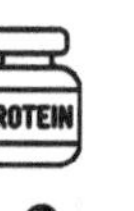 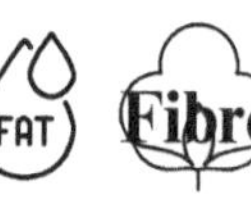 

Prep		CARB	KCAL	PROTEIN	FAT	Fibre	Servings
5 mins	3 mins	41g	162 Cal	1.3g	2g	2.6g	3

Ingredients

- 1 cup of pineapple juice
- 1(15 1/3 ounce) of can fruit cocktail or tropical fruit salad.
- 1 cup non-fat vanilla yogurt
- 1 banana, medium-ripe

Instructions

1. Pour the fruit and juice from the can into a freezer container and either freeze completely or partially.
2. In a blender, combine all ingredients and process until smooth.

Green Goddess Smoothie

 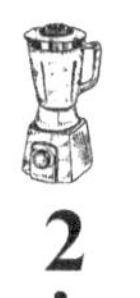 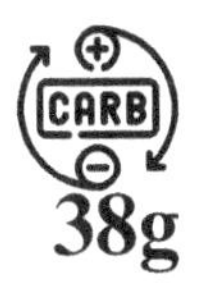  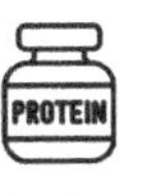 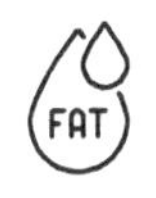 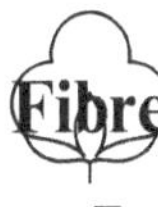 

Prep		CARB	KCAL	PROTEIN	FAT	Fibre	Servings
10 mins	2 mins	38g	198 Cal	1.9g	3g	5g	2

Ingredients

- 1 green apple cored, chopped
- 1/2 small cucumber peeled and chopped
- 3/4 cup fresh spinach
- 1/2 green pear cored, chopped
- 1/2 medium avocado peeled, pitted, and chopped
- 1 peeled kiwi
- 1 scoop vanilla protein powder (optional)
- Water
- Ice cubes

Instructions

1. Put all the ingredients in the listed order into a high-speed blender. To guarantee that everything is combined thoroughly and there are no large pieces of spinach leaves, make sure the spinach is completely overwhelmed by the other ingredients.

2. Process at high speed for 45–60 seconds, or until fully smooth. Sip it from a tall glass.

Pineapple Coconut Smoothie

 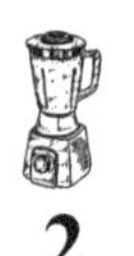 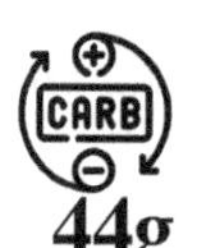  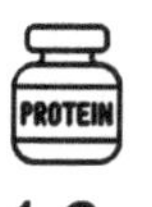 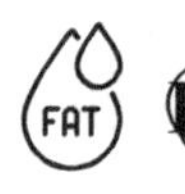 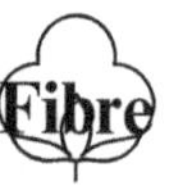 

Prep		CARB	KCAL	PROTEIN	FAT	Fibre	Servings
5 mins	2 mins	44g	403 Cal	4.3g	23g	4.8g	2

Ingredients

- 2 pineapple wedges
- 1 cup coconut milk
- 2 cups of frozen pineapple
- 2 lime wedges
- 1/4 cup sweetened flaked coconut
- 1 banana fresh or frozen
- 2 sprigs of mint
- Garnishes

Instructions

1. In a blender, combine the coconut milk, banana, pineapple, and coconut.
2. Blend until the mixture is very smooth.
3. Dip the rims of two glasses into a plate of coarse sugar and then back into water to garnish them if desired. After adding a mint sprig to each glass, pour the smoothie into them. Arrange a pineapple and lime wedge onto the cup rims.

Minty Matcha Smoothie

 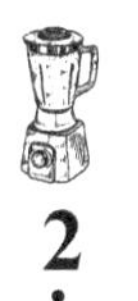 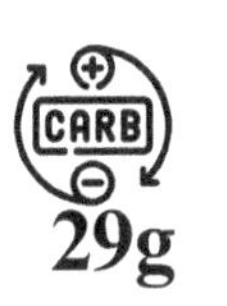 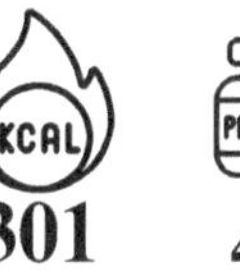 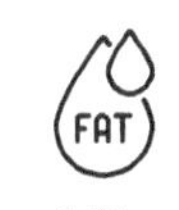 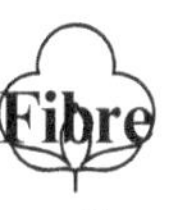 

Prep		CARB	KCAL	PROTEIN	FAT	Fibre	Servings
5 mins	2 mins	29g	301 Cal	4g	17g	6g	2

Ingredients

- 1 cup baby fresh spinach leaves
- 1/4 cup avocado
- 1/2 cup non-dairy milk of choice
- 1 frozen banana
- 1 -2 tablespoons of cacao nibs
- 1 teaspoon of matcha green tea powder
- 1/4 – 1/2 teaspoon of peppermint extract
- 1/2 cup water
- 1/2 cup ice

Instructions

1. In a blender, combine all ingredients except cacao/chocolate; puree until smooth. If more water is required to get the right consistency, add it.

2. Transfer smoothie into container and mix in cacao/chocolate, setting aside a small amount for garnish.

Chocolate Raspberry smoothie

 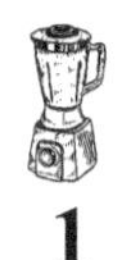 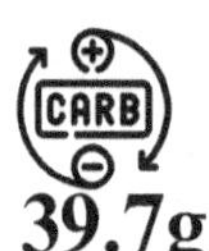 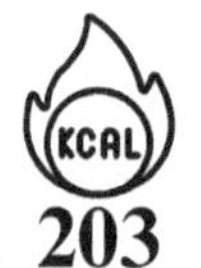 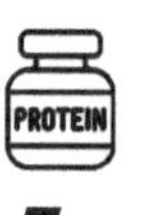 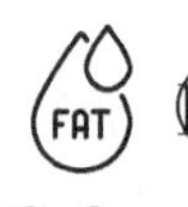 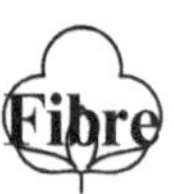 

Prep		CARB	KCAL	PROTEIN	FAT	Fibre	Servings
5 mins	1 mins	39.7g	203 Cal	7g	3.3g	7.3g	2

Ingredients

- 1 cup raspberries
- 1 banana
- 2 tablespoons cocoa powder, unsweetened
- ½ cup of milk
- ½ cup natural yogurt
- 1 tablespoon of honey

Instructions

1. 1.Blend the bananas, milk, yogurt, honey, cocoa powder, and bananas.
2. Blend until a thick, smooth consistency is achieved.
3. Bon Appetit!

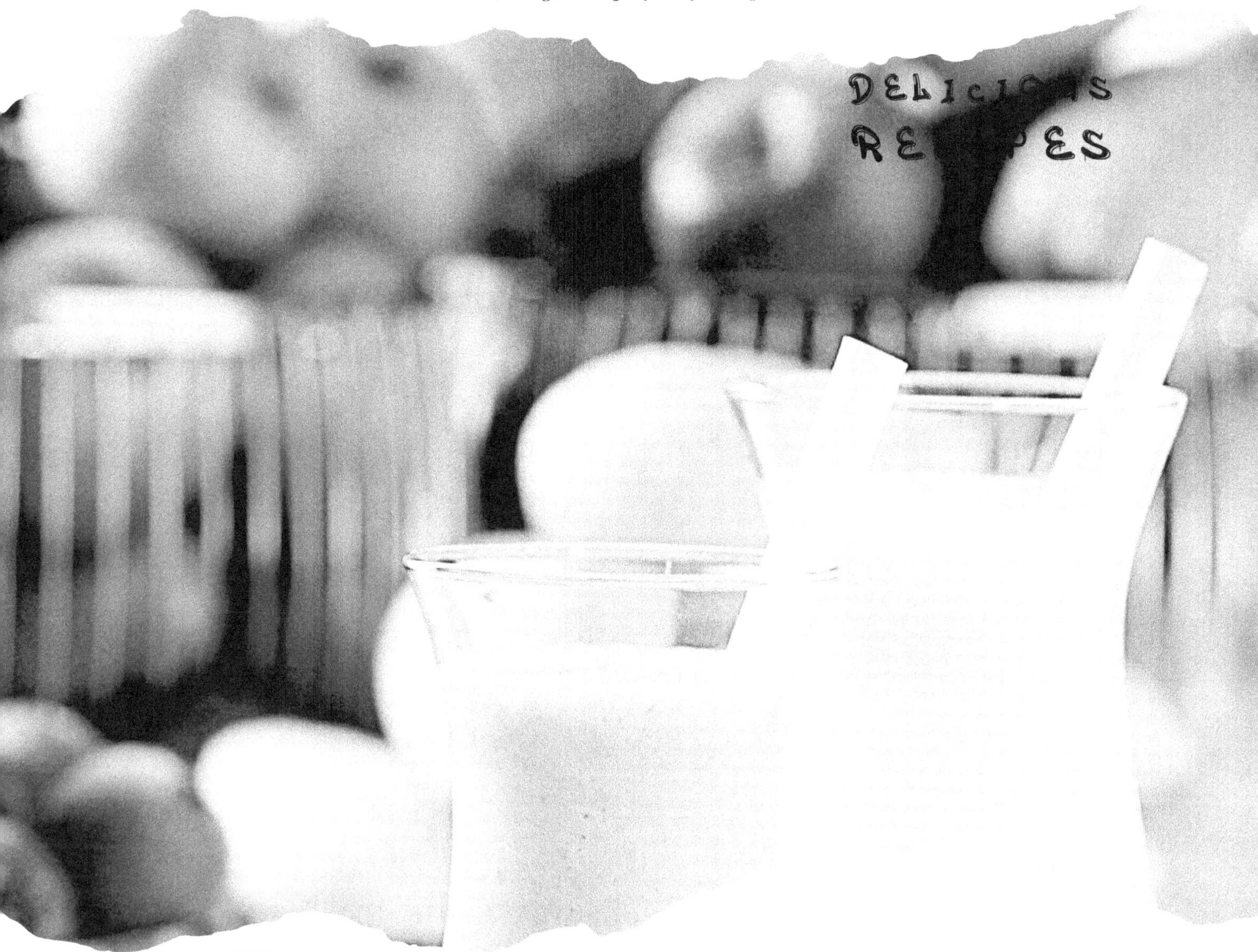

BEVERAGES
RECIPES

—— FOR HEALTHY YOU ——

Green Juice

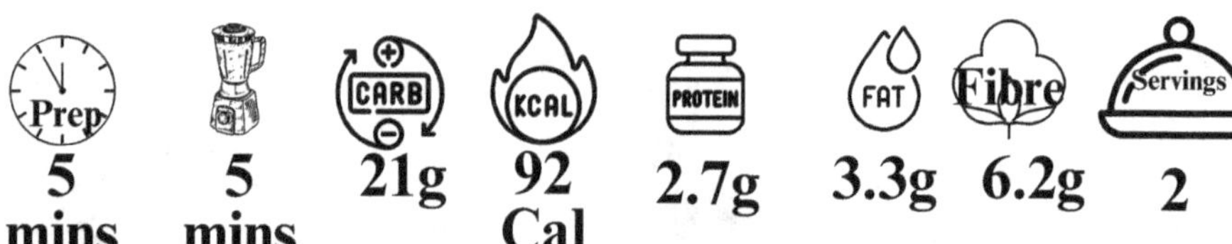

Prep		CARB	KCAL	PROTEIN	FAT	Fibre	Servings
5 mins	5 mins	21g	92 Cal	2.7g	3.3g	6.2g	2

Ingredients

- 1 bunch kale (about 5 ounces)
- 1 inch peeled fresh ginger
- 1 Granny Smith apple (or large apple)
- 5 stalks of celery, ends trimmed
- ½ large cucumber
- A handful of fresh parsley (about 1 ounce)

Instructions

1. Clean and ready the veggies.
2. Cut it into large pieces. juice according to the prescribed order. (Or, use a blender to blend it.)
3. Pour the green juice into a glass if using a juicer, and serve right away.
4. The juice will thicken when you use a spoon. Transfer into a fine-mesh strainer and press the flesh into the strainer with the back of a spoon to extract as much liquid as you can.
5. Enjoy the filtered juice after pouring it into the glass!

Kale Juice

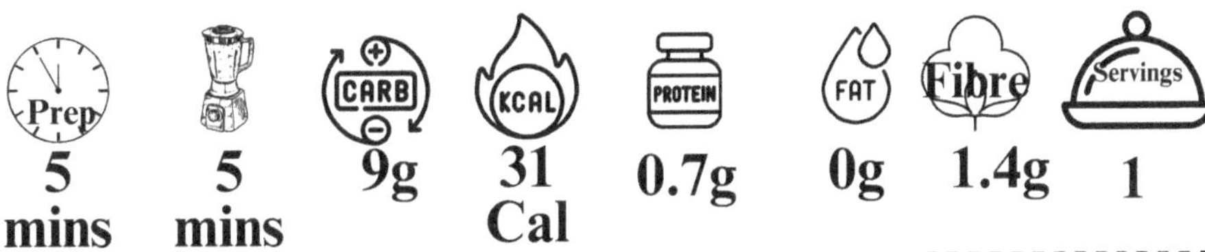

Prep		CARB	KCAL	PROTEIN	FAT	Fibre	Servings
5 mins	5 mins	9g	31 Cal	0.7g	0g	1.4g	1

Ingredients

- 1 bunch kale
- 1 cucumber
- 1 1-inch piece of fresh ginger
- 1 green apple
- 1 lemon, peeled
-

Instructions

1. After washing, pat dry the kale leaves.
2. Dice the cucumber and apple into small enough pieces to pass through the feeding tube of your juicer.
3. Next, switch on your juicer. Put all of the ingredients, including the stems and leaves of the kale, into the juicer. To get the best performance out of the juicer, alternate between hard and soft ingredients.

Turmeric Latte

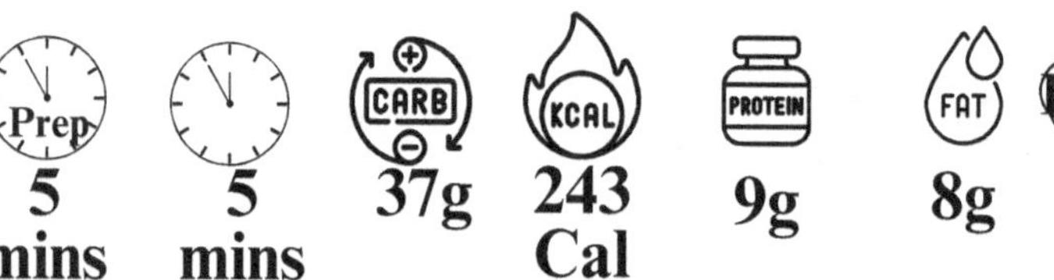

Prep		CARB	KCAL	PROTEIN	FAT	Fibre	Servings
5 mins	5 mins	37g	243 Cal	9g	8g	1g	1

Ingredients

- 1/2–1 tsp agave nectar or other natural sweetener
- 1 1/4 cups plain, unsweetened nondairy milk
- Grated fresh ginger, 1/2 teaspoon
- 1/8 tsp ground cinnamon,
- 1/4 tsp ground turmeric, and 1/8 tsp ground cardamom, optional
- 1/2 tsp vanilla extract(optional)
- 1/16 tsp black pepper, roughly a pinch
- 1/16 tsp cayenne pepper,(optional)

Instructions

1. Transfer the soy milk into a tiny saucepan and set it over medium heat.
2. In order to loosen up any remaining spice clumps, thoroughly whisk in the agave, fresh ginger, turmeric, cinnamon, cardamom, black pepper, and cayenne.
3. Make sure not to let the mixture boil as you gently simmer it for two to five minutes.
4. Warm up after pouring into a mug.

Matcha Tea

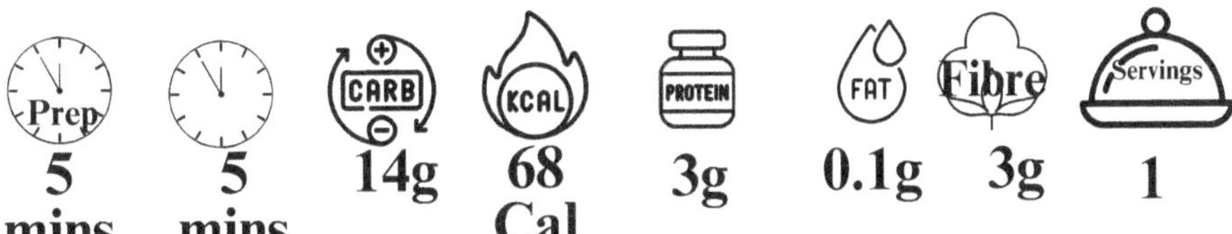

Prep		CARB	KCAL	PROTEIN	FAT	Fibre	Servings
5 mins	5 mins	14g	68 Cal	3g	0.1g	3g	1

Ingredients

- ½ to 1 teaspoon matcha powder
- ¼ cup hot water
- ¼ cup coconut milk, warmed
- Honey, stevia, or sweetener of choice, optional

Instructions

1. Pour the matcha into a large mug after straining it to remove any lumps, then quickly whisk in an up-and-down motion until it foams, which should take about 30 seconds.

2. Add the coconut milk and whisk again until thoroughly mixed.

3. Taste and adjust the amount of water, coconut milk, and/or sweetener to your preference.

Cucumber Mint Cooler

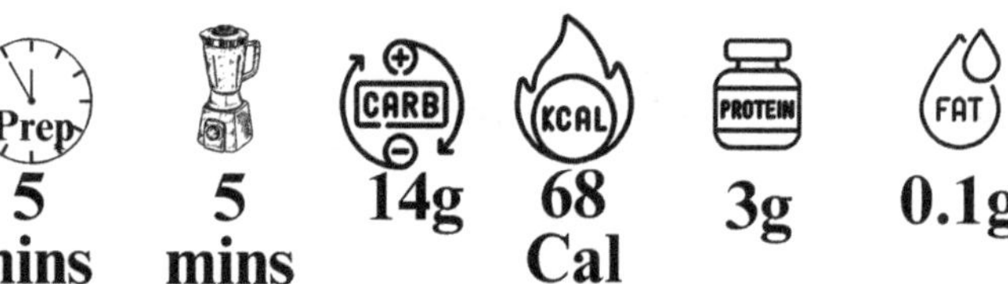

Prep		CARB	KCAL	PROTEIN	FAT	Fibre	Servings
5 mins	5 mins	14g	68 Cal	3g	0.1g	3g	1

Ingredients

- Fresh mint leaves
- 1 green apple, sliced and cored
- 2 handfuls of ice
- 1/4 cup 100% pure honey
- 1 sliced cucumber
- 1 cup of cold water
- 2 tablespoons of lime juice

Instructions

1. In the specified order, add the ingredients to a high-speed blender and process until smooth.
2. Add the mint leaves at this time if you plan to grind them into the beverage. Add the leaves to the finished drink, if infusing, and chill for a few hours before serving.
3. Take the leaves off before consuming.
4. Refrigerate for two to three days.

Berry Juice

 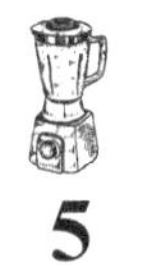 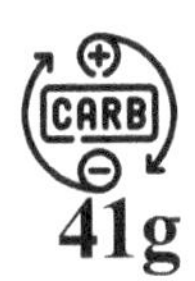  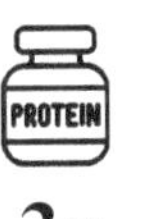 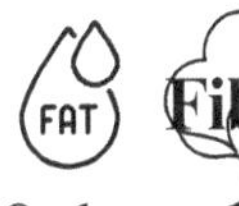 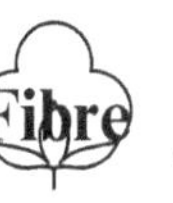 

Prep		CARB	KCAL	PROTEIN	FAT	Fibre	Servings
5 mins	5 mins	41g	192 Cal	3g	0.1g	14g	1

Ingredients

- 1 cup strawberries, hulled, cut in quarters
- 1 cup pineapple, cut in 1-inch pieces
- 1 orange, peeled, cut in quarters
- 1/2 cup blueberries
- 1/2 cup raspberries

Instructions

1. Place ingredients into the feed chute in the specified order after pressing START/STOP. Don't load more into the feed chute until the juicer has finished processing every piece for optimal results. Press ingredients through the feed chute with the pusher as necessary.

Watermelon Mint Refresher

 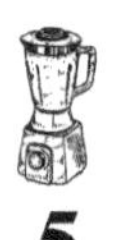 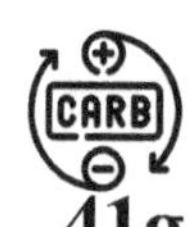  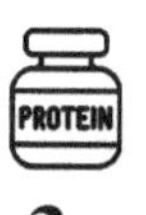 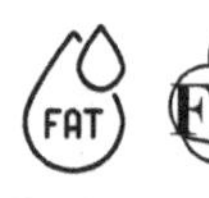 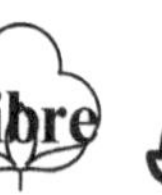 

Prep		CARB	KCAL	PROTEIN	FAT	Fibre	Servings
5 mins	5 mins	41g	192 Cal	3g	0.1g	14g	1

Ingredients

- 2 cups watermelon chunks
- 4-5 ice cubes
- 2 fresh mint leaves
- 1/2 tsp agave
- 1/4 cup water
- few squeezes of fresh lime juice

Instructions

1. Blend all ingredients together in a high-speed blender until smooth.

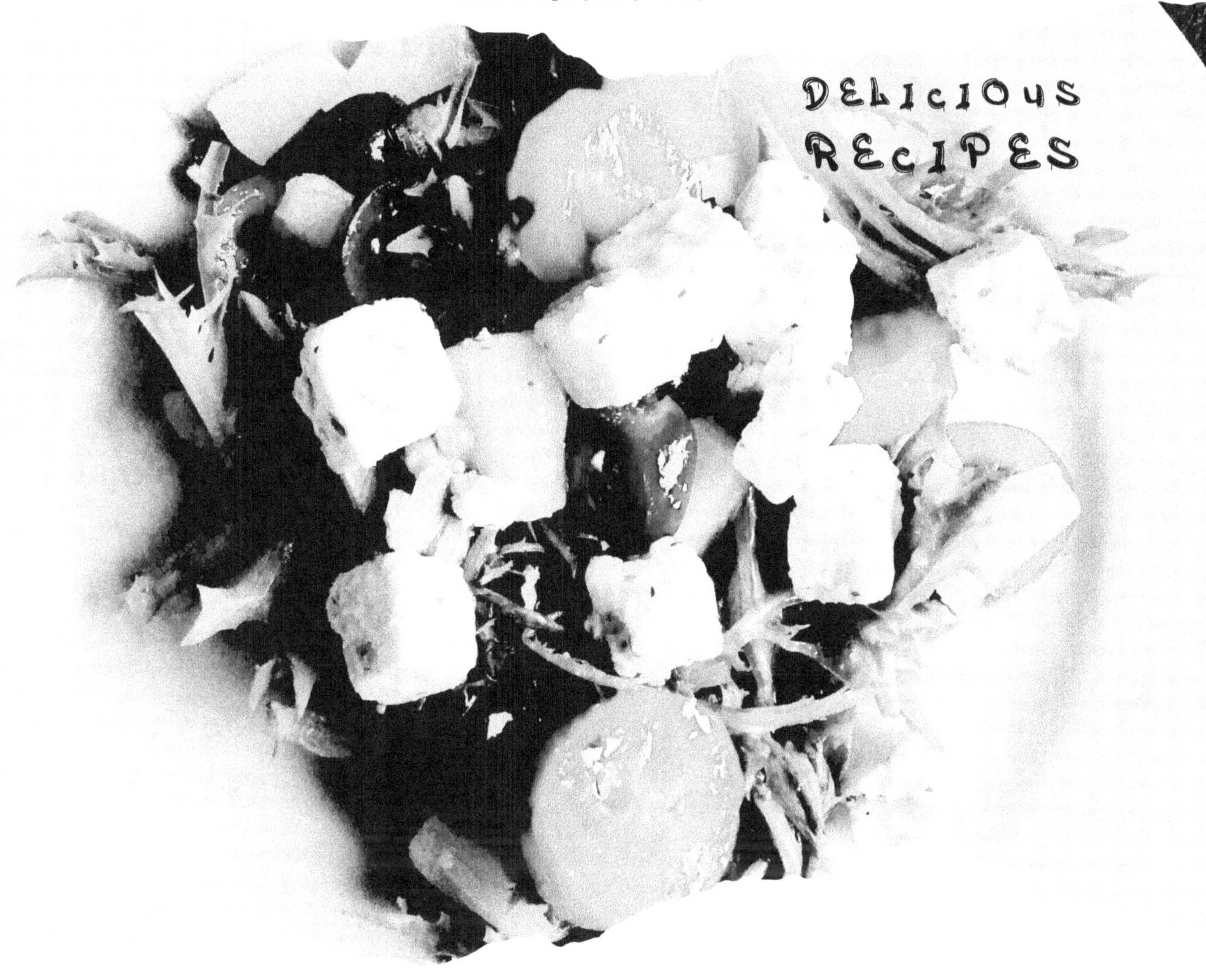

SALADS

RECIPES

—— FOR HEALTHY YOU ——

Caprese Salad

 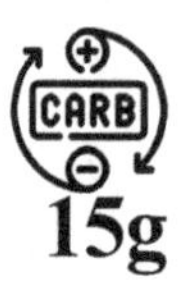  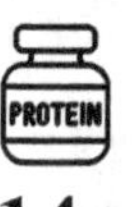 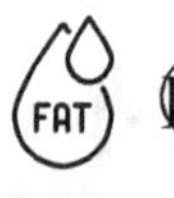 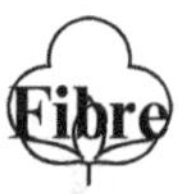 

Prep	CARB	KCAL	PROTEIN	FAT	Fibre	Servings
5 mins	15g	261 Cal	14g	20g	1g	6

Ingredients

- 1 bunch fresh basil
- 1½ pounds ripe tomatoes
- 3 tablespoons olive oil
- Freshly cracked black pepper
- Salt
- 2 tablespoons balsamic glaze
- 12-16 ounces fresh mozzarella

Instructions

1. Arrange tomato slices in layers on a serving platter. Place cheese slices so that they are visible between each tomato, and then place whole basil leaves between the cheese and the tomatoes. Orient the slices so that each layer is visible.

2. Add as much salt and pepper to taste, and generously drizzle with extra virgin olive oil and two tablespoons of balsamic glaze.

Tuna Nicoise Salad

 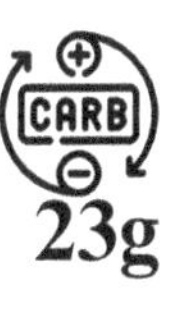  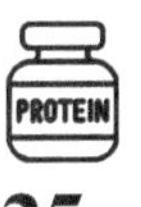 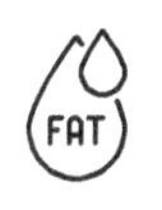 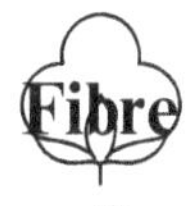 

Prep	CARB	KCAL	PROTEIN	FAT	Fibre	Servings
5 mins	23g	334 Cal	25g	16g	0g	4

Ingredients

- 100g fresh baby salad
- 450g waxy potatoes, thickly sliced and not peeled.
- 4 eggs.
- 50g sundried tomato in oil, chopped.
- 1/2 red onion, sliced thinly.
- 2 x 160g or 200g cans yellowfin tuna steak in springwater, drained
- 2 tsp olive oil.
- 1 tablespoon of red wine vinegar.
- 2 tablespoon caper, rinsed.

Instructions

1. Preheat the oven to 200°C, 180°C for the fan, and 6°G. Add a little oil (2 tsp) and seasoning to the potatoes. Transfer to a sizable baking sheet and bake for 20 minutes, flipping once, or until thoroughly cooked, golden, and crispy.

2. In the meanwhile, crack the eggs into a small pan of water, bring to a boil, and simmer for 8 to 10 minutes, depending on your preference for doneness. To cool off for a short while, submerge yourself in a bowl of cold water. Before cutting into halves, remove the shells.

3. Combine the chopped tomatoes, red wine vinegar, capers, and remaining oil in a sizable salad bowl. After adding the potatoes, tuna, onion, and spinach, season and toss gently. Add the eggs on top, then serve immediately.

229

Greek Salad

 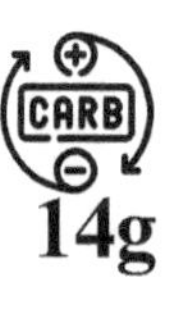 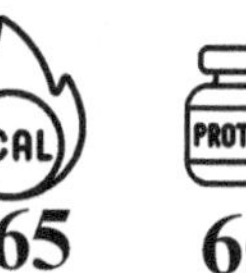 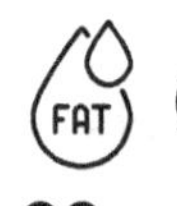 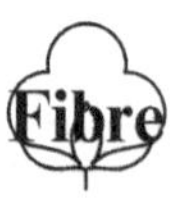 

Prep	CARB	KCAL	PROTEIN	FAT	Fibre	Servings
20 mins	14g	265 Cal	6g	22g	3g	6

Ingredients

- 1 head of romaine lettuce – rinsed, dried and finely chopped
- 1 cucumber, thinly sliced
- 2 large tomatoes, chopped
- 1 (6 ounce) pitted black olives
- 1 green pepper, chopped
- 1 red pepper, finely chopped
- 1 red onion, thinly sliced
- 1 cup crumbled feta cheese
- 6 tablespoons of olive oil
- 1 lemon, juice and preparation
- 1 teaspoon dried oregano
- Ground black pepper to taste

Instructions

1. Romaine, cucumber, tomato, olives, green pepper, and red onion should all be combined in a big bowl. Add some feta cheese on top.
2. Mix the lemon juice, olive oil, oregano, and pepper in a small bowl.
3. Drizzle the salad with the vinaigrette, toss to coat, and serve.
4. Drizzle the salad with the vinaigrette, toss to coat, and serve.

Asian Sesame Chicken Salad

 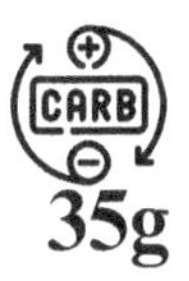  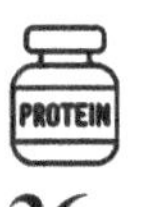 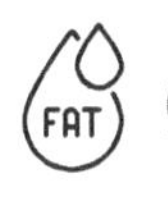 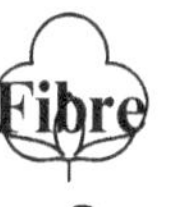 

Prep	CARB	KCAL	PROTEIN	FAT	Fibre	Servings
17 mins	35g	516 Cal	36g	31g	2g	4

Ingredients

Sesame Vinaigrette:

- 1 tablespoon toasted sesame oil and seeds
- ½ cup rice vinegar
- 2 tablespoons soy sauce
- ¼ cup avocado oil
- 2 whole cloves garlic, smashed

Salad:

- ⅓ cup sliced almonds
- 12 ounces grilled chicken, diced or shredded
- 1 large carrot, shredded
- 1 cup prepared wonton strips
- 6-7 cups shredded romaine or baby spinach
- 1 can mandarin oranges, drained
- ½ cup cilantro leaves

Instructions

1. In a small saucepan, combine the rice vinegar and water over medium heat; bring to a gentle boil. Add the garlic cloves about 1 minute. Remove from the stove and discard the garlic cloves. Transfer the rice vinegar mixture to a mason jar; add the sesame oil, canola oil, soy sauce, and sesame seeds; allow the dressing to come to room temperature, about 10-15 minutes. Cover the jar and shake to blend the ingredients; if the dressing separates, shake again.

2. All of the salad ingredients—aside from the wonton strips—should be combined in a big bowl. Add the sesame vinaigrette on top and toss to mix. Add wonton strips on top, then serve right away.

231

Mediterranean Quinoa Salad

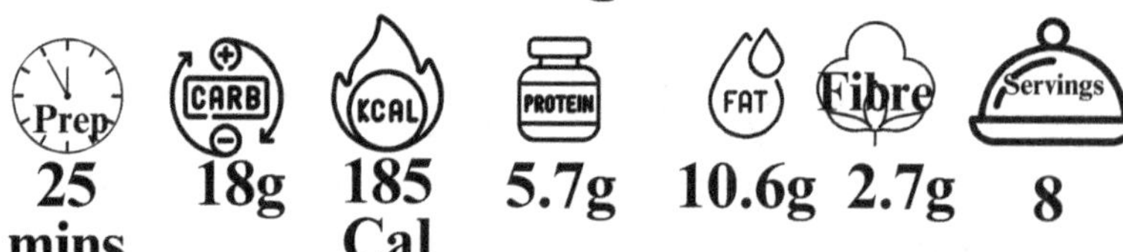

Prep	CARB	KCAL	PROTEIN	FAT	Fibre	Servings
25 mins	18g	185 Cal	5.7g	10.6g	2.7g	8

Ingredients

- 1 cup quinoa
- 1 English cucumber
- 2 bell peppers
- ¼ teaspoon black pepper
- ½ cup crumbled feta cheese
- ¼ cup extra virgin olive oil
- ¾ teaspoon kosher salt
- ½ cup pitted Kalamata olives, drained
- 4 scallions
- 1 teaspoon oregano
- 1 lemon

Instructions

1. Give the quinoa a thorough rinse with cold running water. Cook in accordance with the directions on the package.

2. In a serving bowl, combine the oregano, salt, pepper, and lemon zest and juice while the quinoa cooks. Stir in the extra virgin olive oil. To suit your taste, adjust the seasoning.

3. Add the cooked quinoa to the bowl along with the dressing once it's soft. In order to let the quinoa absorb the lemon dressing, stir to coat. Before adding the vegetables, let it cool completely.

4. Slice and trim the scallions, chop the peppers, and cut the olives into smaller pieces with your knife. Halve the cucumber, then cut it into quarters, and then slice. Pour in the bowl and mix. Add the feta last, then serve.

Avocado Shrimp Salad

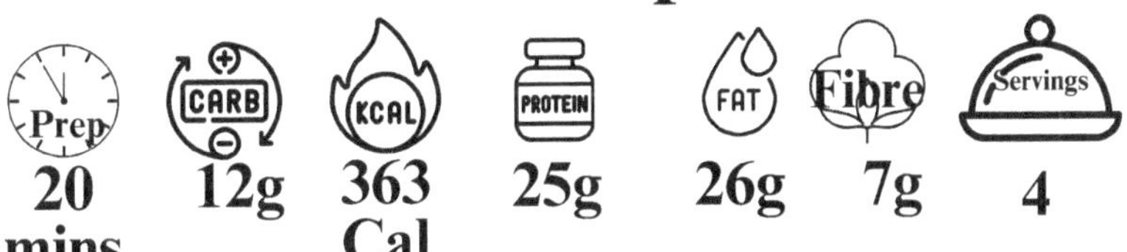

| 20 mins | 12g | 363 Cal | 25g | 26g | 7g | 4 |

Ingredients

- 2 avocados sliced
- 1 pound large shrimp thawed
- ¼ red onion diced
- 2 cups shredded lettuce
- 1 tablespoon chopped cilantro

Dressing:

- 1/2 teaspoon fresh cracked pepper
- 3 tablespoons lime juice
- 1/2 teaspoon salt
- 1 teaspoon cumin
- 3 tablespoons extra-virgin olive oil

Instructions

1. Heat up a big pot of water until it boils. Reduce the temperature to medium. Put the shrimp in a mesh strainer or steamer insert over the water in the pot and cover it with a lid. Steam for 4–6 minutes, or until the shrimp curl and turn bright pink. Take out and place somewhere to cool.

2. Use a bowl big enough to accommodate all the salad ingredients when preparing the dressing. To create an emulsified mixture, whisk together the olive oil, lime juice, cumin, salt, and pepper.

3. Transfer the steaming shrimp to the dressing's surface. Toss in the red onions and shredded lettuce, then mix with the dressing in the bowl. Add some fresh cilantro as a garnish and tuck the sliced avocados around the shrimp.

233

Grilled Chicken Caesar Salad

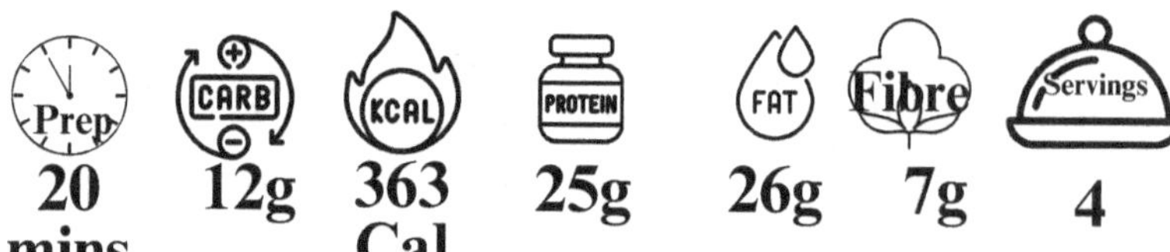

Prep	CARB	KCAL	PROTEIN	FAT	Fibre	Servings
20 mins	12g	363 Cal	25g	26g	7g	4

Ingredients

- 1 ¼ lb boneless chicken breasts
- 2 tablespoons red wine vinegar or lemon juice
- 2 tablespoons olive oil
- ½ teaspoon garlic powder
- ½ teaspoon dried thyme
- ½ teaspoon dried oregano
- ¼ teaspoon salt
- ¼ teaspoon pepper
  SALAD
- Sourdough Croutons
- Caesar Dressing
- 1 head romaine lettuce, chopped into bite-sized pieces
- Fresh parmesan, shaved

Instructions

1. In a small bowl, thoroughly mix vinegar, oil, thyme, oregano, garlic powder, salt, and pepper.
2. Chicken should be put in a shallow dish or a 1-gallon plastic bag that can be sealed. Toss to coat, add the marinade, and chill for a minimum of 1 hour and a maximum of 12 hours.
3. Bake sourdough croutons.
4. Make dressing by blending all the ingredients together until smooth and creamy.
5. Take the chicken out of the marinade, shake off any excess, and discard any marinade that remains. Turn on the grill pan. When the grill is hot, add the chicken and cook it for about five minutes on each side. The internal temperature of the chicken should be 165°F.
6. To assemble the salad, fill two bowls with a bed of romaine lettuce. Add the shaved parmesan, sourdough croutons, and sliced chicken breast. Enjoy after drizzling with Caesar dressing!

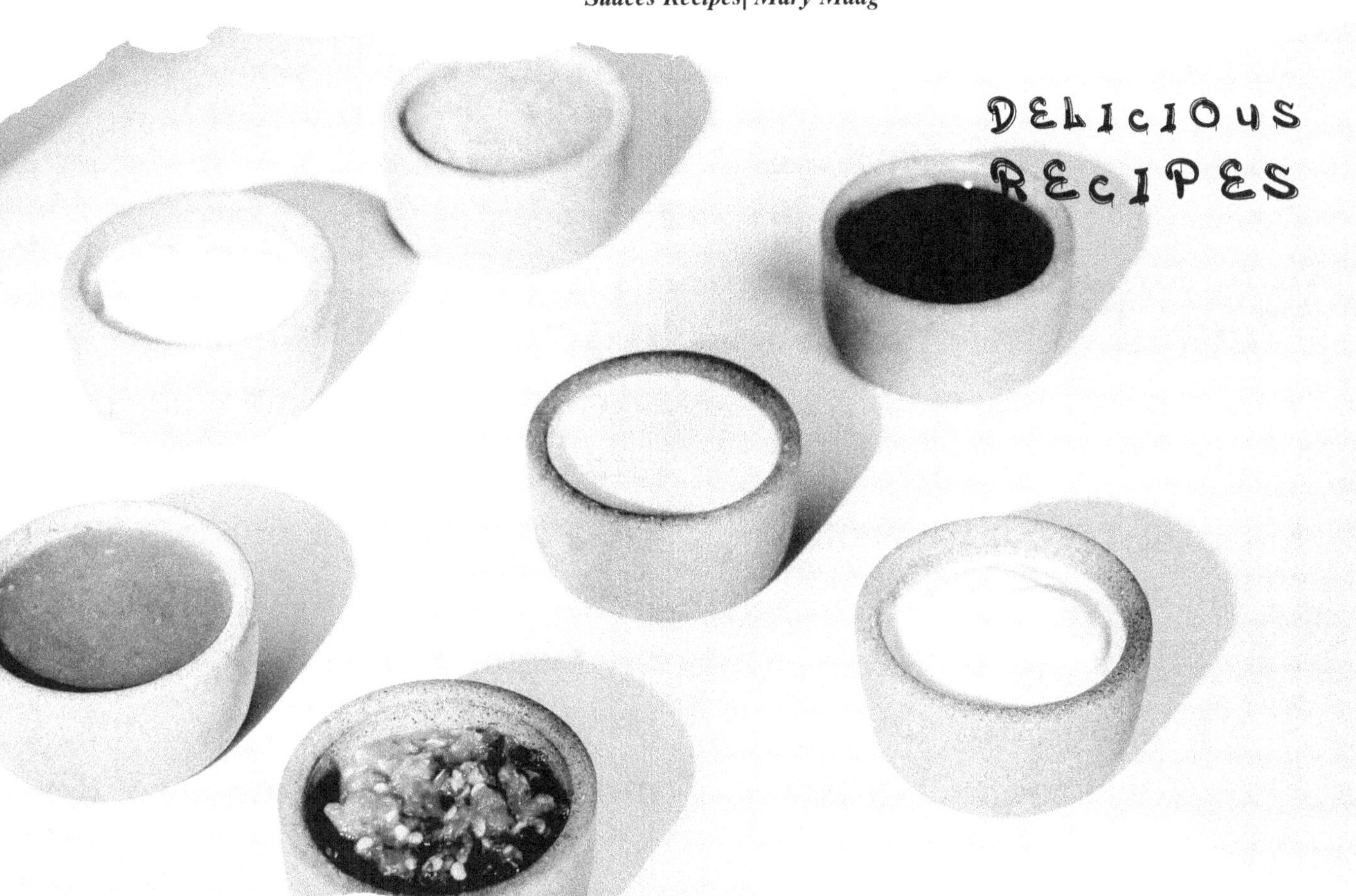

SAUCES & CONDIMENTS RECIPES

—— FOR HEALTHY YOU ——

235

Chimichurri Sauce

 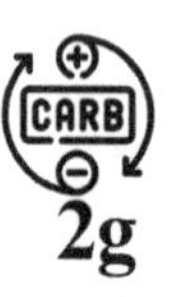  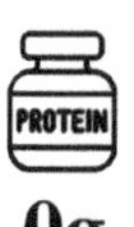 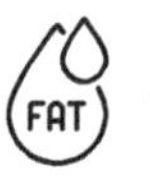 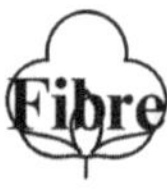 

Prep	CARB	KCAL	PROTEIN	FAT	Fibre	Servings
15 mins	2g	70 Cal	0g	6g	0g	16

Ingredients

- ⅓ cup extra-virgin olive oil
- 2 tablespoons white wine vinegar
- 1 garlic clove, minced
- ½ teaspoon sea salt
- ¼ teaspoon dried oregano
- ¼ teaspoon red pepper flakes
- ¼ teaspoon smoked paprika
- ½ cup finely chopped fresh flat-leaf parsley

Instructions

1. Mix the olive oil, vinegar, garlic, salt, white wine vinegar, oregano, red pepper flakes, and smoked paprika in a small bowl; stir in the parsley. Alternatively, use a mortar and pestle or a food processor for a few quick pulses to combine the ingredients.

2. Season to taste and serve as a sauce for roasted or grilled vegetables.

Sesame Ginger Sauce

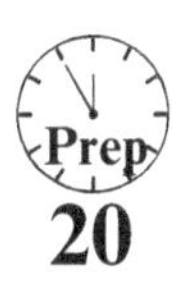 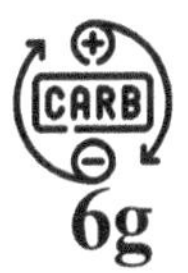  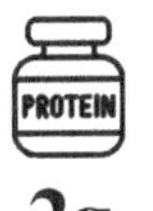 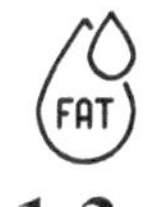 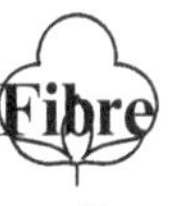 

Prep	CARB	KCAL	PROTEIN	FAT	Fibre	Servings
20 mins	6g	44 Cal	2g	1.3g	0g	1

Ingredients

- 1 teaspoon grated fresh ginger root
- 1 tablespoon Dijon mustard
- 2 ½ teaspoons water
- 1 tablespoons soy sauce
- ¼ teaspoon sesame oil

Instructions

1. Mix the water, ginger root, sesame oil, mustard, and soy sauce in a small bowl and stir.

Coconut Curry Sauce

 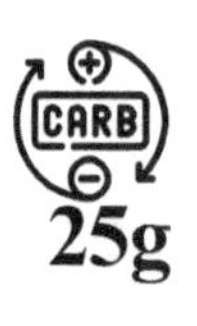 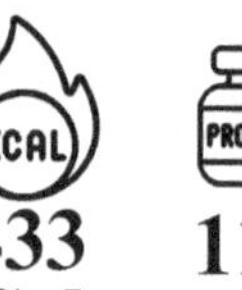 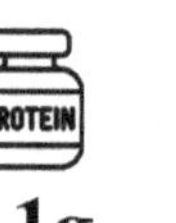 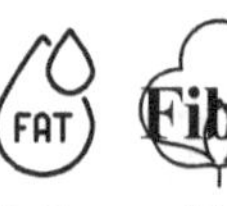 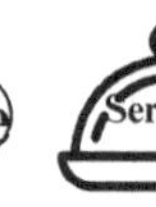 

Prep	CARB	KCAL	PROTEIN	FAT	Fibre	Servings
30 mins	25g	433 Cal	11g	36g	7.3g	4

Ingredients

- 400g/14 Oz can of coconut milk
- 400 g/14 Oz can brown drained lentils
- 80g 2 cups baby spinach
- 1/2 cup cashews
- 2 tsp grated fresh ginger
- 400 g/14 oz can of drained brown lentils
- 1/2 cup tomato puree
- 8 oz pumpkin
- 2 tbsp vegetable oil
- 4 minced garlic cloves
- 1/2 chopped onion
- 1/2 tsp each salt and pepper
- 1 tsp coriander powder
- 1/2 tsp turmeric
- 1 tbsp garam masala
- 2 tbsp curry powder
- 2 tsp cumin
- 1 tsp paprika
- tsp coriander powder

Instructions

1. In a deep skillet or pot, heat the oil over medium-high heat. Add the onion, garlic, and ginger, and cook for 2 minutes, or until the onion begins to turn golden.

2. If the mixture appears a little dry, don't worry. Add the spices and stir for one minute.

3. Add the broth, passata, and coconut milk. Mix until well combined.

4. Add the pumpkin and lentils. After bringing to a simmer, adjust the heat to a vigorous simmer.

5. Simmer for ten minutes, or until the sauce has thickened and the pumpkin is soft but not mushy.

6. After the baby spinach has wilted, stir in the cashew nuts.

7. Finally, add the salt and pepper, tasting as you go.

238

Avocado Cream Sauce

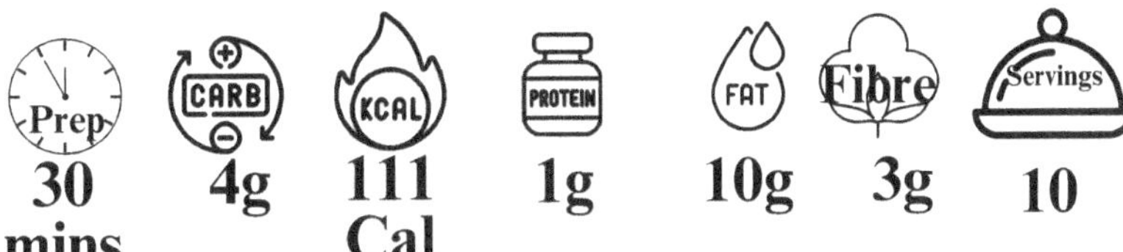

Prep	CARB	KCAL	PROTEIN	FAT	Fibre	Servings
30 mins	4g	111 Cal	1g	10g	3g	10

Ingredients

- 2 large ripe avocados pitted and halved
- 2 large cloves minced garlic
- 1 cup of greek yogurt or sour cream
- 1/8 teaspoon freshly ground black pepper
- ¼ teaspoon kosher salt adjusted to taste
- 3-4 tablespoons of lime juice

Instructions

1. In a blender, combine the avocado, yogurt, garlic, and lime juice; process until fully smooth, and taste and adjust with salt and pepper.

2. Move to a platter and serve right away, or cover tightly with an airtight lid after pressing plastic wrap against the sauce's surface.

3. If you can make the sauce last that long, it will keep well in the refrigerator for up to 48 hours.

Roasted Red Pepper Sauce

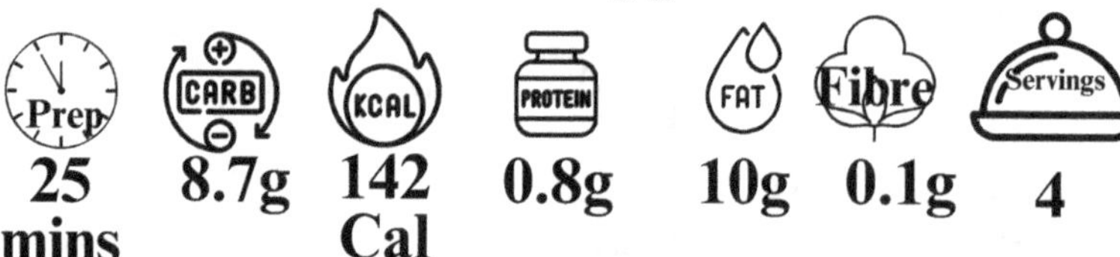

Prep	CARB	KCAL	PROTEIN	FAT	Fibre	Servings
25 mins	8.7g	142 Cal	0.8g	10g	0.1g	4

Ingredients

- 4 cloves of garlic
- Freshly cracked black pepper
- 1/2 teaspoon of dried basil
- 1 16 Oz. jar roasted red peppers
- 1/2 cup heavy cream
- 2 tablespoon of butter

Instructions

1. Place about 2 tablespoon of the jar's liquid in a blender with the roasted red peppers. Blend the peppers until smooth, adding a tablespoon or two of water if necessary to facilitate the puréeing process (don't add too much jar liquid)
2. Add the minced garlic to a skillet along with the butter. The garlic should be softened and fragrant after one to two minutes of medium-low heat sautéing in butter (but not browned). Add the dried basil, freshly cracked pepper, and the puréed peppers. Mix to blend.
3. Let the sauce to simmer for a while. Reduce the heat to low and simmer the sauce, stirring frequently, for ten to fifteen minutes, or until the mixture thickens.
4. When the sauce is smooth, add the heavy cream to the skillet and heat it through.

Basil Pesto

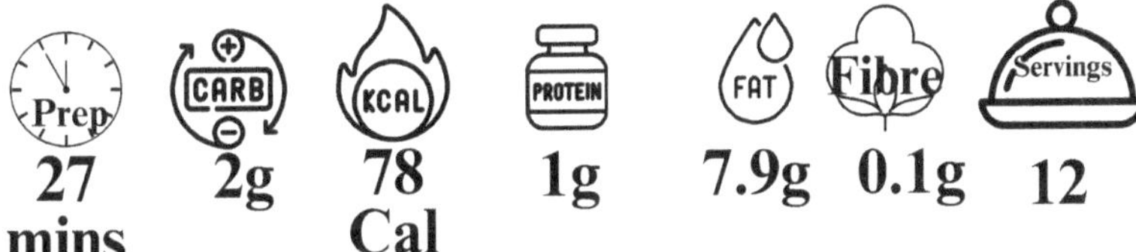

Ingredients

- 2 cups fresh basil leaves (you can use half a basil leaf with baby spinach)
- 1/2 cup (about 2 ounces) freshly grated Romano or Parmesan cheese
- 1/2 cup extra virgin olive oil
- 1/3 cup pine nuts (you can add chopped walnuts)
- 3 garlic cloves, chopped (about 1 tablespoon)
- 1/4 teaspoon salt or more to taste
- 1/8 teaspoon freshly ground black pepper (or more, to taste)

Instructions

1. In the bowl of a food processor, combine the pine nuts and basil, and pulse several times.
2. Repeatedly mix in the garlic and Parmesan or Romano cheese.
3. Using a rubber spatula, scrape down the food processor's sides. Olive oil should be added gradually, in tiny streams, while the food processor is operating. To help emulsify and keep the olive oil from separating, add it gradually while the machine is operating.Stop the food processor occasionally so you can scrape down the sides.
4. Add salt and freshly ground black pepper to taste.
5. Toss as a basic sauce with pasta, spoon over baked potatoes, or serve with toast or crackers.

241

Balsamic Glaze

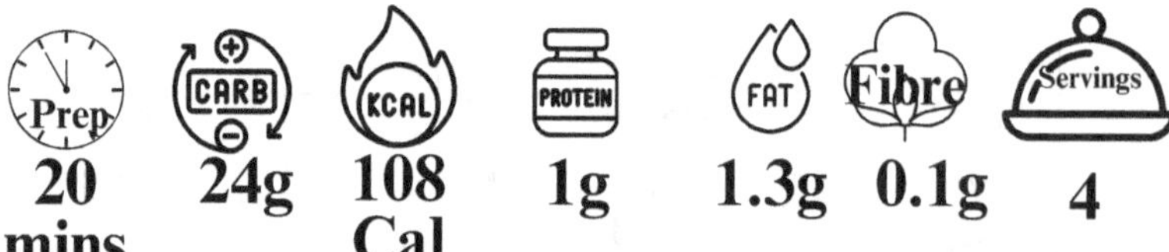

Prep	CARB	KCAL	PROTEIN	FAT	Fibre	Servings
20 mins	24g	108 Cal	1g	1.3g	0.1g	4

Ingredients

- 1/4 cup brown sugar
- 1 cup balsamic vinegar

Instructions

1. In a small saucepot, combine the brown sugar and balsamic vinegar. To dissolve the sugar, stir.
2. Increase the heat to medium and bring the mixture to a simmer. After lowering the heat to medium-low and simmering the mixture for a while with frequent stirring, you should have roughly half of its original volume. This should take about ten minutes, may vary. When the bubbling vinegar thickens to the point where it stays on the surface rather than instantly bursts, you know it's done.
3. After taking the glaze off the stove, let it cool. It will solidify significantly more when it cools. Simmer it one more time if too thick. You can thin the glaze with a tiny bit of water if it's too thick.
4. After cooling, pour the glaze over your preferred dishes and savor! Store leftovers in the refrigerator for up to three weeks or until needed.

Tzatziki Sauce

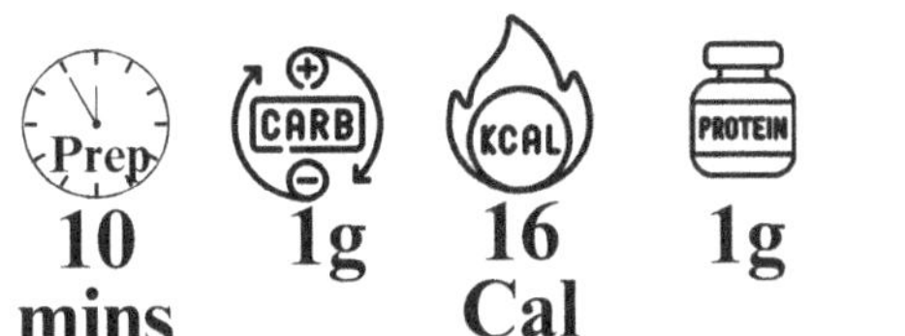

Prep	CARB	KCAL	PROTEIN	FAT	Fibre	Servings
10 mins	1g	16 Cal	1g	0.7g	0.1g	2

Ingredients

- 2 cups plain Greek yogurt
- 4 to 5 minced garlic cloves
- ¼ teaspoon ground white pepper
- 1 teaspoon kosher salt, divided
- 1 tablespoon Extra Virgin Olive Oil
- Handful of chopped fresh dill or mint (optional)
- 1 teaspoon white vinegar
- ¾ English cucumber, peeled
- Warm pita bread for serving
- Sliced vegetables for serving

Instructions

1. Grate the cucumbers by hand using a box grater. Add ½ teaspoon of kosher salt to the grated cucumbers and toss. Grate the cucumber and transfer it to a cheesecloth or two-layered napkin, then squeeze out any excess moisture.
2. Combine the garlic, extra virgin olive oil, white vinegar, and the remaining ½ teaspoon salt in a large mixing bowl. Toss to blend.
3. To the bowl containing the garlic mixture, add the grated cucumber. Add the yogurt, fresh herbs, and a dash of either white or black pepper. Stir well.
4. Before serving, cover and chill for a while (anywhere from 30 minutes to a few hours). This will allow the flavors to meld together and help give the sauce the best texture and thickness.
5. When it's time to serve, give the tzatziki sauce a quick stir, then transfer it to a serving bowl and top with extra virgin olive oil, if desired. Serve alongside your preferred vegetables.

Sriracha Mayo

 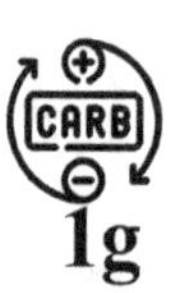  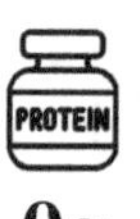 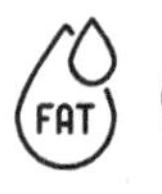 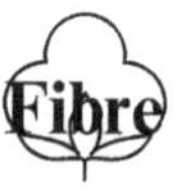 

Prep	CARB	KCAL	PROTEIN	FAT	Fibre	Servings
10 mins	1g	102 Cal	0g	11g	0.1g	16

Ingredients

- ¼ cup Sriracha sauce
- 1 cup mayonnaise
- 1 teaspoon ground black pepper
- ½ tablespoon lemon juice

Instructions

1. In a bowl, thoroughly mix mayonnaise, Sriracha, lemon juice, and black pepper. Serve right away or store in the fridge.

Guacamole

 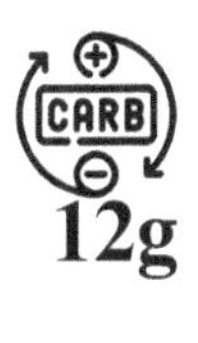  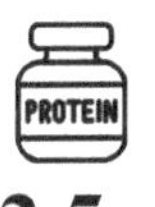 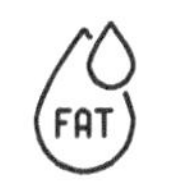 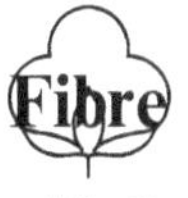 

Prep	CARB	KCAL	PROTEIN	FAT	Fibre	Servings
10 mins	12g	184 Cal	2.5g	15.6g	7.6g	4

Ingredients

- 3 Ripe avocados
- ½ finely diced small yellow onion
- 2 Roma tomatoes
- 3 tablespoons of chopped fresh cilantro
- 1 jalapeno pepper, seeds removed and diced
- 2 minced garlic cloves
- 1 lime, juiced
- ½ teaspoon sea salt

Instructions

1. Divide or slice the avocados, remove the pit, and scoop the flesh into a mixing bowl.
2. Using a fork, mash the avocado until it's as smooth or chunky as you desire.
3. Stir together after adding the remaining ingredients. Taste it and adjust with a little more salt or lime juice.
4. Serve and enjoy!

This page was intentionally left blank.

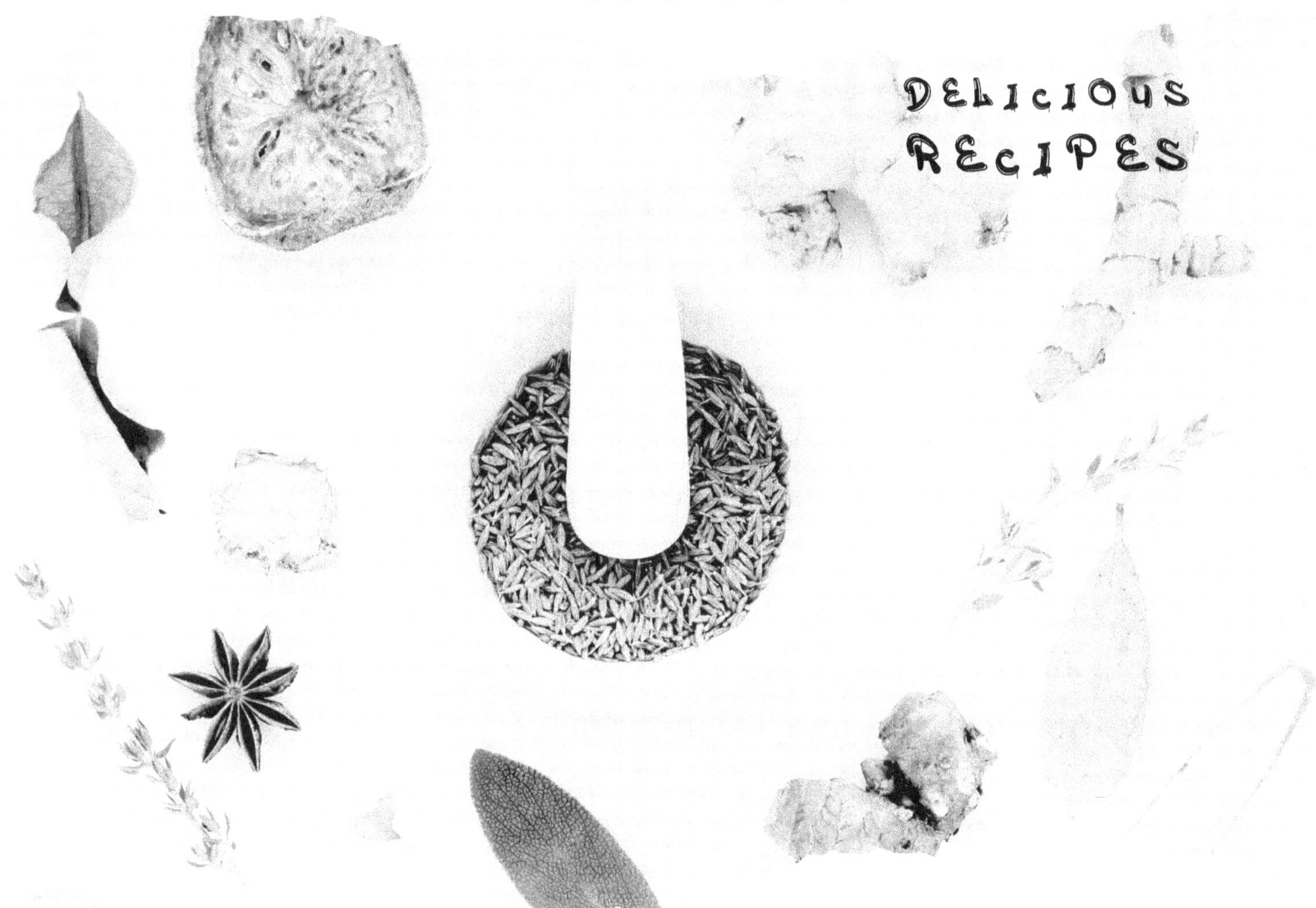

BUYING OF ORGANICS

—— FOR HEALTHY YOU——

Buying Of Organics

Organic products are becoming increasingly popular in our contemporary world, where concerns about sustainability and health are paramount. Regardless of your experience with food shopping or familiarity with living without pesticides, it's important to know how to make an informed decision when choosing what product is best for you and your family.

This chapter's goal is to arm you with helpful knowledge and helpful shopping tips so you can confidently navigate the organic aisle. Together, you and I can enhance your family's health by interpreting or dissecting the labels on significant purchases.

Organic Labels

Numerous products will have "organic" labels when you go shopping for grocery in your favorite super market. Have you ever wondered how to interpret the contents of these letters and what they mean?

Making informed decisions for the environment, your family's health, and your health is dependent on your understanding of organic labels. This quick guide will assist you in deciphering product labels and making an informed decision about which product best suits your needs and the needs of your family.

Types of organic labels

In the grocery store, you can find a variety of organic labels. This label offers details on organic certification and production methods and is subject to regulations. These are a few examples of organic types:

1. "100% organic":

According to this label, there are no synthetic or non-organic ingredients in the product because it is made entirely of organic ingredients. The label requires that only organic ingredients be used in products.

2. "Organic":

"Organic" products have to have at least 95% organic ingredients. The remaining 5% may or may not include non-organic ingredients, which are frequently challenging to grow organically.

3. "Made with organic ingredients":

Products with at least 70% organic ingredients are eligible to use this label. It still means that it uses key organic ingredients even if the product itself doesn't meet the 95% requirement for the "organic" label.

4. "Verified Non-GMO Project":

The Non-GMO Project Verified label, while not organic, certifies that a product is free of genetically modified organisms (GMOs). Since the use of artificial sweeteners is forbidden in organic production, this label is also present on a large number of organic products.

5. "Organic USDA":

Among the most recognizable organic labels is the United States Department of Agriculture's (USDA) Organic Seal. There are numerous variations.

Products labeled as "100% organic" are made entirely of organic ingredients. Products are considered "organic" if at least 95% of their ingredients are organic.

Products labeled as "Made with organic ingredients" have at least 70% organic ingredients.

6. "Certified Organics[Certification Body]":

Numerous certification bodies with USDA approval can certify people on their own. This document certifies that the product has undergone testing in accordance with organic standards.

7. "Biodynamic":

By stressing agricultural integration and sustainability, biodynamic agriculture goes beyond organic practices. Products that are certified by Demeter International are frequently linked to biodynamic products.

8. "Fair Trade Certified":

This certification denotes that a product satisfies specific social, economic, and environmental requirements; it is not just about organic practices. Additionally, some organic products might bear this label.

Guide for Shopping Organic Produce

Purchasing organic goods can involve considerations for one's health as well as emotions. This guide will assist you in selecting organic products with knowledge.

1. Recognizing the organic label:
Watch out for labels claiming to be organic, such as "made with organic ingredients," "100% organic," and "organic." The percentage of organic content in each product is displayed on the graph.

2. Examine certification seals:
Seek out certifications from organizations that certify organic products, such as "USDA Organic." These seals serve as proof

that the product has undergone organic processing.

3. Prefer seasonal and local goods:

Select seasonal, organic, locally grown produce. Seasonal produce is fresher and tastes better, and local produce may have a smaller carbon footprint.

4. Go shopping at the farmer's market:

Make direct connections with nearby growers and producers by going to farmers' markets. This enables you to inquire about the farm and guarantee that the products you purchase are fresh, local, and primarily organic.

5. Examine the following Community Supported Agriculture (CSA) program:

You can obtain fresh, organic food straight from nearby farms by signing up for a CSA program. They also support regional agriculture.

6. Bulk purchases:

Think about purchasing organic basics in large quantities, such as grains, legumes, and nuts. This lowers the amount of waste produced and can be cost-effective in the long term.

7. Examine the list of ingredients:

It's crucial to read the ingredient list, even for organic products. There's still a chance that some processed foods have extra sugar, preservatives, or other non-organic ingredients.

8. Choose the entire menu:

Select unprocessed, organic, whole foods. The best options for a nutritious diet are lean meats, whole grains, fresh produce, and vegetables.

9. Examine Meat and Dairy Alternatives That Are Organic:

Select meat substitutes and dairy products that are organic if you have a vegetarian or vegan diet. When purchasing meat products, look for labels such as "Organic Grass-Fed".

10. Search for Verification of Non-GMO:

In addition to organic certification, look for products bearing the "Non-GMO Project Verified" label if you value avoiding genetically modified organisms (GMOs).

11. Verify Expiration Dates:

Because organic products don't contain preservatives, their shelf lives may be shorter. Plan your purchases by keeping an eye out for expiration dates.

12. Examine Prices:

Even though organic products can cost more, shop around and think about spending your money on the organic products that are most important to you, like those on the Dirty Dozen list.

13. Keep Up with the News:

Keep up with issues pertaining to organic farming and current organic standards. Understanding the organic market can help you make more thoughtful decisions.

14. Promote Open Brands:

Choose businesses with transparent ethical sourcing and production practices.

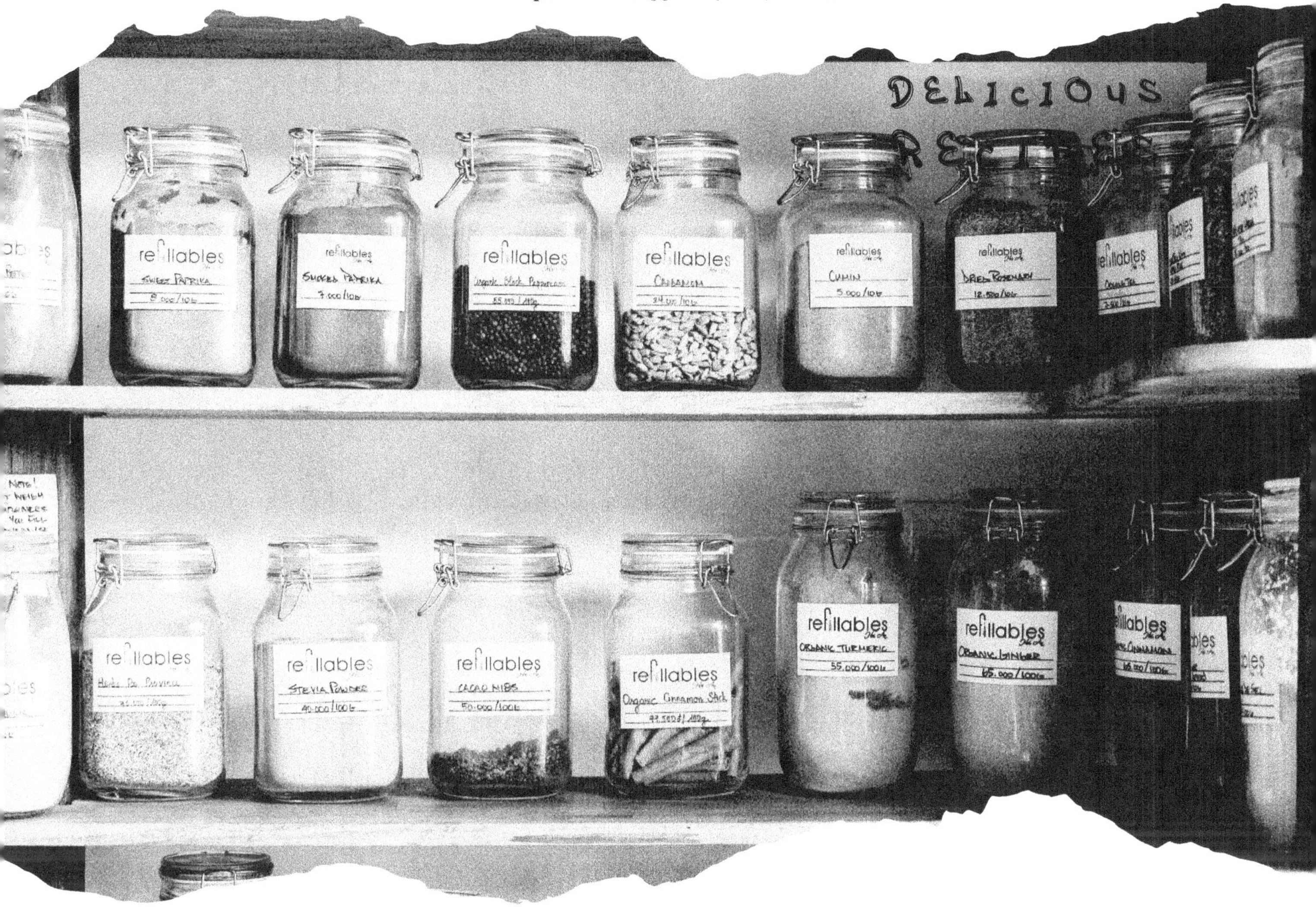

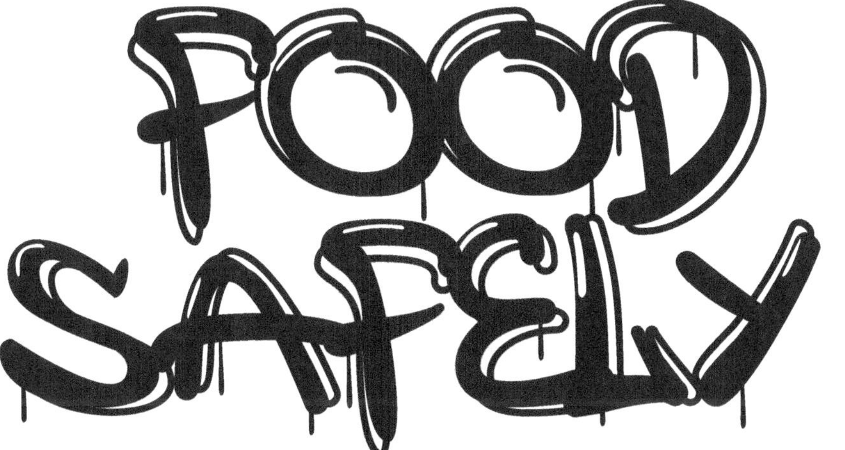

STORING YOUR
FOOD SAFELY

FOR HEALTHY YOU

Advice For Food Preservation

Beyond just knowing how to cook, maintaining the freshness and quality of your food is essential to improving health and cutting waste. Preserving pantry staples, perishables, and leftovers can all be greatly enhanced by adhering to sensible food storage guidelines. You can keep the best ingredients on hand by following these helpful suggestions:

1. Temperature Matters:

To inhibit the growth of bacteria, keep your refrigerator at the recommended temperature, which is less than 40°F or 4°C. For best freezing, maintain your freezer at 0°F (-18°C).

2. Safely Store Raw Meats:

To avoid cross-contamination, store raw meats on the lowest shelf in the refrigerator. To catch any juices, put them in leak-proof containers.

3. Airtight Containers for Perishables:

Use airtight containers to keep perishables like fruits, vegetables, and leftovers fresh.This prevents odors from spreading and prolongs the freshness of items.

4. Use clear containers: Whenever feasible, choose transparent containers. This makes it easier for you to see what's inside, which lessens the chance that something will be wasted or forgotten.

5. First In, First Out (FIFO):

Use the pantry and refrigerator as examples of the FIFO method. To minimize food waste and keep older items from expiring, use them first.

6. Properly Package Freezer Items:

To avoid freezer burn, use freezer-safe bags or containers when freezing food. Put the date on the item for convenient tracking.

7. Label and Date Containers:
Write the date of preparation or purchase on the labels. This is particularly important for products with a short shelf life and leftovers.

8. Eggs Should Be Refrigerated:
Eggs should be refrigerated to maintain freshness. Store them in the original carton to guarantee preservation of quality and protection.

9. Organize your supplies:

Keep your supplies neat and grouped together by similar items. Regularly check the dates on the packaging, and throw away any stale or expired goods.

10. Frequently and thoroughly clean Check Refrigerator: Ensure that spills and expired goods are removed from your refrigerator on a regular basis. Inspect the food for indications of spoilage and make any necessary temperature adjustments.

11. Prevent Overcrowding:

Make sure the pantry and refrigerator have enough air to circulate. Food freshness may suffer from uneven cooling caused by overcrowding.

12. Divide Large Portions: Divide up large quantities of leftover food into smaller containers. This encourages faster cooling while preserving quality.

13. Dark and Cool Storage for Pantry Goods:

To maintain the quality of your pantry goods, store them in a cool, dark place. Keep them out of the heat and direct sunlight.

14. Make Good Use of Produce Drawers:

Make use of your refrigerator's designated produce drawers.

To accommodate various fruit and vegetable varieties, they frequently feature humidity settings that can be adjusted.

15. Rotate Stock Frequently:
To make sure that older items are used first, rotate the stock in your pantry and refrigerator on a regular basis. This keeps things from unintentionally expiring.

Reducing Food Wastage

Approximately one-third of the food produced worldwide is wasted due to a variety of factors. This comes to about 1.3 billion tons annually.

The Recycle Track System (RTS) estimates that 2.5 billion tons of food are wasted globally each year, with the US throwing away more food than any other nation at a rate of almost 60 million tons, or $218 billion, annually. According to estimates, this accounts for approximately 40% of the US food supply, or 325 pounds of waste per person. It's similar to tossing over 900 oranges in the trash can.

Even though these numbers might seem overwhelming, you and I can stop this destructive behavior by adhering to a few straightforward suggestions, which include:

1. Plan Your Meals Ahead of Time: Set aside some time to schedule all of your meals for the coming week. Preparing this ahead of time lowers the likelihood that perishable foods will spoil before you use them and helps you purchase only the groceries you need.

2. Make a Grocery List: Based on the meals you have planned, make a thorough list of everything you need before heading to the grocery store. Adhere strictly to your shopping list to prevent impulsive purchases of unnecessary items.

3. Become knowledgeable about expiration dates: Discover how to distinguish between "sell by," "use by," and "best before" dates. Recognize that these are not hard deadlines, but rather recommendations for when freshness peaks.

4. First In, First Out (FIFO): Make use of your pantry and refrigerator's FIFO system. To keep older items from expiring without your knowledge, use them first.

5. Appropriate Food Storage: To extend the shelf life of fruits, vegetables, and perishable goods, store them properly. Make use of produce drawers, airtight containers, and appropriate storage settings.

6. Use Leftovers Creatively: To cut down on the likelihood of leftovers going uneaten, get creative with them and incorporate them into new recipes or the next day's meal.

7 Freeze extra produce: Before it goes bad, freeze any extra fruits, vegetables, or herbs that you don't need. Frozen produce can be used in soups, smoothies, and other recipes down the road.

8. Recycle Food Scraps: Gather materials such as coffee grounds, fruit cores, and vegetable peelings and start a compost bin. In addition to reducing landfill waste, composting improves soil.

9. Pay attention to portion sizes: When cooking, pay attention to portion sizes. If you're still hungry after eating smaller portions at first, go back for seconds or drink more water because most times we mistake thirst for hunger.

0. Donate Unused Non-Perishable Foods: During your weekly pantry purge, consider donating any unopened non-perishable items that you probably won't use. Such donations are gladly accepted by many food banks.

11. Rejuvenate Wilted Fruit:Bring back the crispness and usability of wilted vegetables and herbs by soak them in ice.

12. Understand Appropriate Food Storage: Recognize which foods are best kept in a cool, dark pantry or in the refrigerator.

13. Utilize Every Part of the Produce: You can use the peels and stems of broccoli and citrus fruits to make coleslaw.

14. Purchase perishables Considerately: Estimate how much you can use before perishables go bad. If the items have short shelf lives, steer clear of buying in bulk.

DAY 11

☐ **Breakfast**

Quinoa Breakfast Bowl

☐ **Lunch**

Pizza Salad

☐ **Dinner**

Turkey and Vegetable Stir-Fry with Brown Rice

DAY 12

☐ **Breakfast**

Spinach and Mushroom Frittata

☐ **Lunch**

Salmon Quinoa Bowl

☐ **Dinner**

Pasta Carbonara with Crispy Kale

DAY 13

☐ **Breakfast**

Brown Rice Pancake

☐ **Lunch**

Adzuki Sandwich

☐ **Dinner**

Spicy seafood

DAY 14

☐ **Breakfast**

Cherry Scones

☐ **Lunch**

Grilled Chicken Salad

☐ **Dinner**

Baked Salmon with Quinoa and Steamed Asparagus

DAY 15

☐ **Breakfast**

Broccoli Feta Frittata

☐ **Lunch**

Shrimp and Avocado Sushi Bowls

☐ **Dinner**

Fish Tacos

DAY 16

☐ **Breakfast**

Pear Rosemary Bread

☐ **Lunch**

Grilled Veggie and Hummus Wrap

☐ **Dinner**

Lemon ginger Salmon

DAY 17

☐ **Breakfast**

Maple Sausage Scramble

☐ **Lunch**

Baked Falafel

☐ **Dinner**

Spring pesto pasta

DAY 18

☐ **Breakfast**

Scrambled Eggs with Zucchini

☐ **Lunch**

Lamb meatball

☐ **Dinner**

Shrimp and Veggie Skewers with Quinoa Tabbouleh

DAY 19

☐ **Breakfast**

Omelette with Vegetables

☐ **Lunch**

Asian Beef and Broccoli Stir-Fry

☐ **Dinner**

Lasagna

DAY 20

☐ **Breakfast**

Smoked Salmon and Avocado Toast

☐ **Lunch**

Tomato Greek salad

☐ **Dinner**

Moroccan Lamb Tagine

DAY 21

☐ **Breakfast**

Quinoa Breakfast Bowl

☐ **Lunch**

Pizza Salad

☐ **Dinner**

Turkey and Vegetable Stir-Fry with Brown Rice

DAY 22

☐ **Breakfast**

Spinach and Mushroom Frittata

☐ **Lunch**

Salmon Quinoa Bowl

☐ **Dinner**

Pasta Carbonara with Crispy Kale

DAY 23

☐ **Breakfast**

Brown Rice Pancake

☐ **Lunch**

Adzuki Sandwich

☐ **Dinner**

Spicy seafood

DAY 24

☐ **Breakfast**

Cherry Scones

☐ **Lunch**

Grilled Chicken Salad

☐ **Dinner**

Baked Salmon with Quinoa and Steamed Asparagus

DAY 25

☐ **Breakfast**

Broccoli Feta Frittata

☐ **Lunch**

Shrimp and Avocado Sushi Bowls

☐ **Dinner**

Fish Tacos

DAY 26

☐ **Breakfast**

Pear Rosemary Bread

☐ **Lunch**

Grilled Veggie and Hummus Wrap

☐ **Dinner**

Lemon ginger Salmon

DAY 27

☐ **Breakfast**

Maple Sausage Scramble

☐ **Lunch**

Baked Falafel

☐ **Dinner**

Spring pesto pasta

DAY 28

☐ **Breakfast**

Scrambled Eggs with Zucchini

☐ **Lunch**

Lamb meatball

☐ **Dinner**

Shrimp and Veggie Skewers with Quinoa Tabbouleh

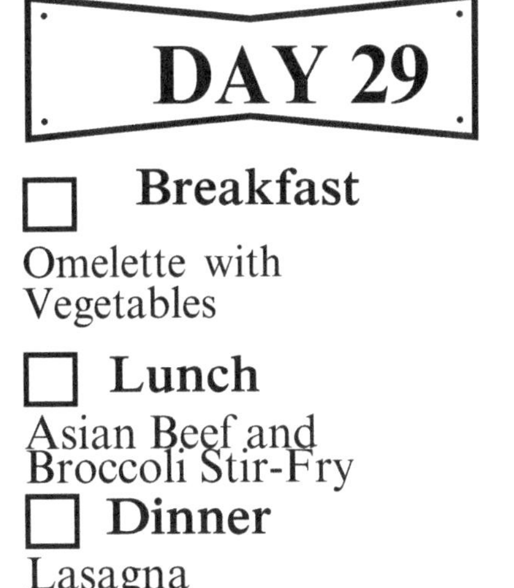

DAY 29

☐ **Breakfast**

Omelette with Vegetables

☐ **Lunch**

Asian Beef and Broccoli Stir-Fry

☐ **Dinner**

Lasagna

DAY 30

☐ **Breakfast**

Smoked Salmon and Avocado Toast

☐ **Lunch**

Tomato Greek salad

☐ **Dinner**

Moroccan Lamb Tagine

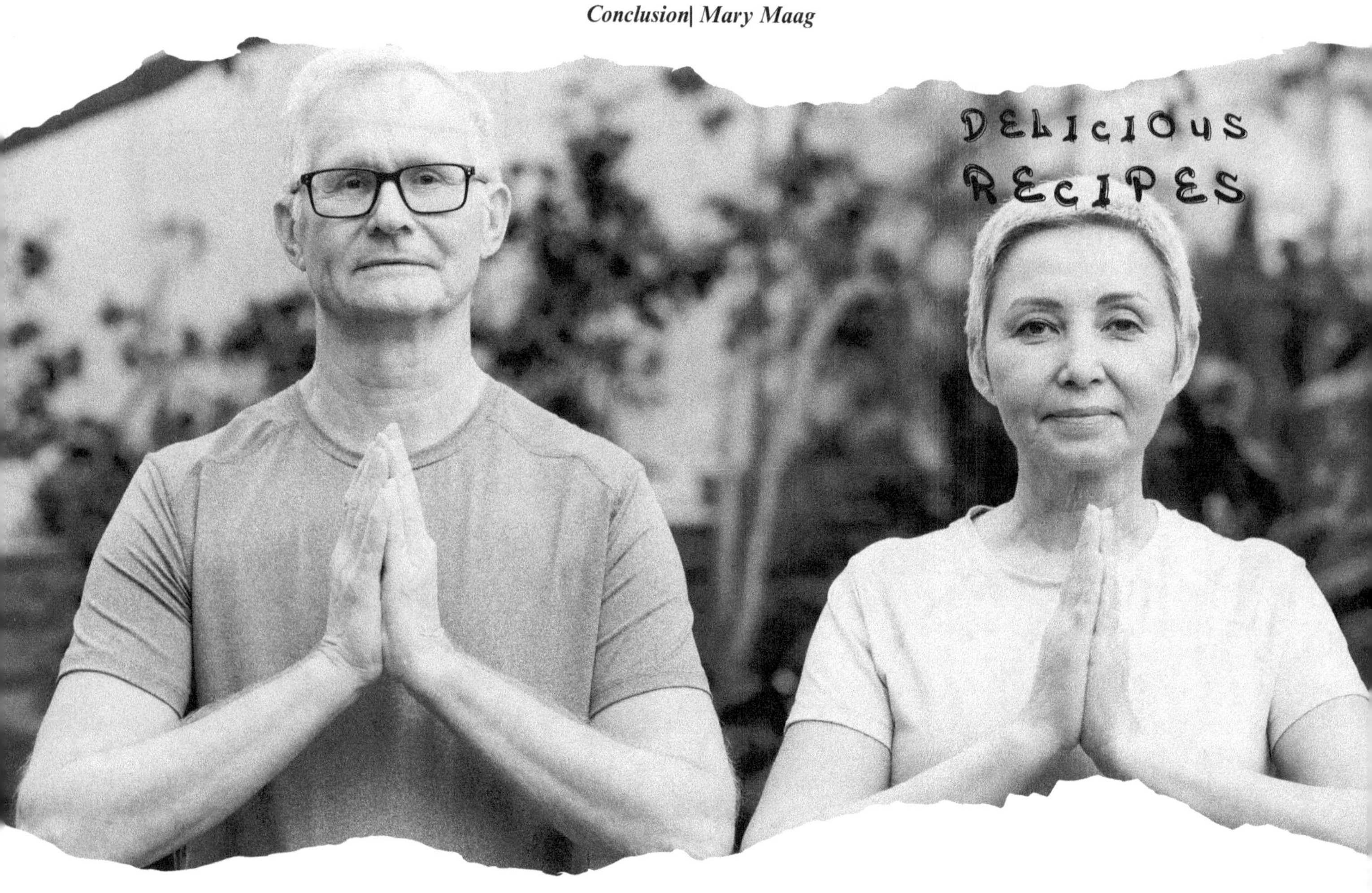

CONCLUSIONS

Let's pause to recap the essential components that have flavored our investigation as we turn the last page on our understanding of the Blood Type O- Negative diet: knowledge, purpose, and the delicious flavors of healthy living.

We've unlocked the mysteries of the Blood Type O- diet through these sections, revealing the balance between your blood type and what your body needs to be fed. You now possess a cooking compass that points you in the direction of a path of vitality and balance, having progressed from understanding the basics to creating delectable recipes customized for your health.

However, this is not where the journey ends; instead, it becomes a dynamic adventure that you, my dear reader, are now prepared to take on. As you approach the brink of transformation, let me urge you to incorporate the knowledge you have acquired into your everyday existence, rather than merely absorbing it.

Highlights summarized:

Customized Diet:
The specific nutritional requirements for your blood type O-are unique. For maximum health benefits, adopt a diet rich in vegetables, lean meats, and specific grains.

Conscious Eating:
Savor every bite, pay attention to your body's cues, and be grateful for the nourishment you give.

Well-Proportioned Recipes:
This book's chapters have revealed a range of recipes for breakfast, lunch, dinner, and delectable snacks. Discover and enjoy the variety of tastes that correspond to your blood type.

- Foods to Steer Clear of:

Avoid foods that might not be as good for your blood type. It's just as important to recognize what you should not do as it is to embrace what makes you feel better.

- Take Action Now and Record Your Cooking Adventure:

Now that you are aware of these guidelines, I urge you to act. Put this knowledge into practice by entering your kitchen with intention and filling your house with the aroma of health-conscious cooking. Don't stop there, though; continue by recording your steps and journey.

Write a journal that distills the essence of your culinary journey. Write down the recipes that end up being your go-to ones, watch for little changes in your energy levels, and share your knowledge with other people who are interested in wellness. By keeping track of your progress, you not only demonstrate your commitment but also contribute to a collective experience that inspires others to pursue well-being.

Recall that the goal is progress, not perfection. Every tiny tweak, every thoughtful decision, is a step closer to being a better, more energetic version of yourself. So open your diary and start writing down not just recipes but also how your health has changed over time.

Dear Esteemed Reader,

As we end this insightful exploration of the Blood Type O– diet, I would like you to share your insightful opinions and experiences with this recipe book. Your input is vital to us as we continue to improve this book.

I would greatly appreciate your thoughts on this joint venture after you have prepared the dishes, followed the instructions, and maybe changed them to suit your needs. Please share what went well, any difficulties you ran into, and any recommendations you might have.

Your experiences can motivate and teach others in our community. I eagerly await your commentary on the recipes, recommendations, and any areas we could expand upon in future editions. Your input steers the direction of this project.

We appreciate your attention to health and willingness to investigate a blood type-specific diet. Your willingness to share your journey with this book advances our collective pursuit of a healthy lifestyle. I'm excited to continue our conversation and use your suggestions to make future editions even better.

To provide feedback, please visit Amazon.com and search Mary Maag, or use the QR code below. Thank You!

Kind wishes,   **Mary Maag**